WHEN WAITING BECOMES LIFE

*Encouraging Stories and Medical Advice
from the Heart of an Infertility Doctor*

JEFF DEATON, MD

LUCIDBOOKS

When Waiting Becomes Life:
Encouraging Stories and Medical Advice from the Heart of an Infertility Doctor
Copyright © 2025 by Jeff Deaton, MD

Published by Lucid Books in Houston, TX
www.LucidBooks.com

ISBN: 978-1-63296-856-2 (Paperback)
ISBN: 978-1-63296-857-9 (Hardback)
eISBN: 978-1-63296-858-6

Special Sales: Most Lucid Books titles are available in special quantity discounts. Custom imprinting or excerpting can also be done to fit special needs. Contact Lucid Books at Info@LucidBooks.com

To Mary
Your unwavering devotion, steadfast love,
and gentle spirit have been the enduring foundation of
my adult life and career.

To Taylor
Your integrity, inquisitive mind, and adventurous spirit
have made me a better person and, more importantly, a
better dad. It has been a profound joy watching the writer
in you awaken the writer in me.

To Eddy
Your perseverance, work ethic, and independent spirit
have enriched one of my favorite roles in life: being a dad.
The resilience you have shown throughout the years has
been a true inspiration to me.

TABLE OF CONTENTS

A WORD FROM DR. DEATON

SPECIAL THANKS

*T*o all the patients, especially those who grace the pages of When Waiting Becomes Life: Your unwavering honesty, immense courage, and remarkable strength continue to be a wellspring of inspiration. Thank you for sharing the most intimate aspects of your lives and for entrusting a young doctor with such a deeply personal journey. It has been an honor to partner with each of you in bringing new life into the world.

To my exceptional colleagues at Wake Forest University and Premier Fertility: Infertility care is, without a doubt, a team sport. I have been immeasurably blessed with the finest teams in all of medicine. Not only did you provide exceptional care and bring thousands of children into the world, but you also infused our work with joy and camaraderie. Thank you for your patience and for the invaluable journey we shared as we learned and grew together.

To the visionaries at Lucid Books: While I may know how to carefully place an embryo into a uterus, I had no idea how to prepare and present my book to the world. Your passion for these stories and your deep love for books were an immense source of encouragement. Without your dedication and talent, *When Waiting Becomes Life* would have remained just an idea in my heart.

In loving memory of Paula and Robin: Your steadfast devotion to me and profound love for our patients were a constant, guiding force at both practices for many years. You truly inspired us all, and your presence in this world was cut short far too soon.

PREFACE

A Note from Dr. Jeff Deaton:

My journey into the world of reproductive medicine began nearly three decades ago, shaped by an inspiring mentor during my time at Vanderbilt University where I completed both my undergraduate studies and medical school. This early guidance led me to pursue a residency in obstetrics and gynecology at the University of Connecticut, followed by a specialized fellowship in reproductive endocrinology and infertility at the University of Vermont.

After my infertility training, I ventured to Winston Salem, North Carolina, to establish the IVF program at Wake Forest University. For 16 years, I poured my energy into building that program, eventually venturing into private practice for a decade with my dedicated team. Today, I'm honored to be back at Wake Forest, directing the Center for Fertility and Reproductive Surgery.

Through 30 years of walking alongside individuals and couples facing infertility, certain profound themes have emerged. First, I've witnessed firsthand the often-hidden shame that can weigh heavily on women who are unable to conceive. This journey is, without doubt, an emotional roller coaster—a complex fusion of raw human emotion, cutting-edge science, and boundless compassion. I've also come to understand the unique and often silent burden carried by the partners of those undergoing treatment. My role has often shifted, requiring me to be a scientist, physician, counselor, financial advisor, and proceduralist, sometimes all at once.

Finally, there's the waiting. This journey is punctuated by an almost constant state of anticipation—waiting for ovulation, waiting for insemination, waiting for egg retrieval, waiting for embryo transfer, and perhaps most acutely waiting for the results of a pregnancy test.

It is for all these reasons—to address the complexities, the emotions, and the unique science—that I wrote this book. My deepest desire is to offer encouragement, hope, and practical advice to couples who are navigating the unique and deeply personal journey of infertility, especially those who cannot visit our practice in person. This book is a distillation of three decades of experience, designed to be a companion as you face one of life's most challenging yet ultimately hopeful paths.

INTRODUCTION

Waiting—we spend a lifetime in its grip, a constant rhythm of anticipation. From the mundane to the momentous, we all carry the quiet hum of something hoped for. Perhaps even now you feel it, the subtle tension of a desired outcome yet to arrive. Within this universal experience, we discover a paradox. Sometimes the crucible of waiting refines us, forging resilience and inner strength whether our deepest desires are met or not. The very act of enduring can make us better.

Yet there are moments when the weight of waiting becomes unbearable when it presses down, suffocating hope, and threatening to isolate us in shadows of depression. For those on the sacred, often agonizing journey to parenthood, this waiting is a unique torment. It is an anxiety unparalleled, a constant echo of "what if?" What if this prolonged hope, this fervent desire, never culminates in the gentle cry of a child? What if, against all odds, the waiting finally yields the longed-for baby? Will this relentless unknown make you more resilient for life's inevitable trials, or will it exact a crushing toll, leading you to withdraw from the very life you yearn to embrace?

Navigating the landscape of infertility can feel like traversing a shadowy and lonely terrain. The path is often fraught with emotional turbulence, medical complexities, and the quiet ache of unfulfilled dreams. For couples yearning to build a family, each month can bring a renewed cycle of hope and disappointment, casting a long shadow over their relationship and their connection with loved ones. The weight of endless appointments, invasive procedures, and the uncertainty of it all can strain even the strongest bonds, leaving individuals and couples feeling lost and misunderstood.

Beyond the medical and emotional hurdles, there is often a heavy burden of unwarranted shame. The intensely personal nature of the experience can lead to feelings of being broken or not measuring up, creating a sense of detachment from friends and family who may not fully grasp the complexities involved. Societal norms often center on the expectation of natural conception, inadvertently amplifying the feelings of inadequacy and failure that can accompany infertility. Sharing struggles can feel vulnerable, and the fear of judgment or unsolicited advice can further deepen the silence. This isolation can compound the emotional distress, making an already challenging journey feel even more lonely and difficult to bear.

Within these pages lies a beacon of hope and understanding. This book gathers the resilient voices of individuals who have walked this challenging path, sharing their deeply personal stories of struggle, perseverance, and ultimately triumph in its many forms. Every story involves real people, real pain, and real emotions. In some stories, the names and some details have been changed to protect confidentiality. In other stories, the patients felt strongly that they should be identified for several reasons, not the least of which is to be a source of hope for others.

Alongside these encouraging narratives, you will find accessible and insightful medical advice, carefully chosen to demystify the often-overwhelming world of infertility treatments and options. You will find advice on when and how to seek help, tips on understanding and fighting the shame that lurks alongside infertility, the science behind the menstrual cycle and in vitro fertilization, and the often-difficult decisions surrounding child-free living versus donor eggs versus adoption. There is a valuable Glossary of Terms right after this introduction that will help you learn the new language of infertility care.

Whether you are a couple actively navigating fertility challenges, a family member or friend seeking to offer meaningful support, or simply someone wanting to understand this often-silent struggle, this book offers a compassionate guide. It is a testament to the strength of the human spirit, a source of practical knowledge, and a reminder that you are not alone on this journey. By weaving together personal experiences and expert guidance, this book aims to empower you with information, uplift your spirits, and foster a greater sense of connection and understanding during this significant chapter of your life. Come walk this journey with an expert who will encourage you and provide valuable information to help you move to the next season of life—triumphant!

GLOSSARY OF TERMS

I know typically the Glossary of Terms goes at the back of the book, but because these terms are so central to these stories, I wanted to include them at the beginning so that access is as easy as possible. Familiarize yourself with these terms and then refer back to them as needed along the way.
—Dr. Deaton

Androgens: The male hormones produced by the testicle, ovary, and adrenal gland, primarily consisting of testosterone and androstenedione.

Anovulation: A condition in which the ovaries do not grow a follicle and release an egg in a routine cyclical manner.

Anti-Müllerian hormone (AMH): The hormone produced by the smaller follicles in the ovary, giving a measure of the number of eggs that might develop with FSH injections during an IVF cycle. Also represents the number of eggs remaining in the ovaries and thus is often referred to as the marker of ovarian reserve.

Antral follicle count (AFC): A diagnostic test that measures the number of small (1–8 mm) follicles in the ovaries at the beginning of a menstrual cycle, providing another indication of ovarian reserve.

Aromatization: The process whereby testosterone is converted to estradiol and androstenedione is converted to estrone. This process is critical in the formation of the dominant follicle each month.

Assisted hatching (AH): A laboratory procedure in which a small opening is made in the outer shell (zona pellucida) of the embryo to help it hatch and implant in the uterine lining.

Assisted reproductive technologies (ART): A general term referring to fertility treatments that involve handling eggs, sperm, or embryos outside the body, including IVF, ICSI, and ZIFT.

Azoospermia: The complete absence of sperm in the ejaculate.

Beta-hCG (human chorionic gonadotropin): A hormone produced during pregnancy. A blood test for beta-hCG is used to confirm pregnancy and monitor its progression.

Blastocyst: An embryo, roughly 120 microns in diameter, which has developed for five to six days after fertilization, consisting of an outer layer of cells (trophectoderm) that will form the placenta, an inner cell mass that will develop into the fetus, an outer shell (zona pellucida), and a cyst cavity.

Cervix: The lower, narrow part of the uterus that connects to the vagina. It consists of an external os that opens into the vagina and an internal os that opens into the cavity of the uterus, thereby allowing sperm to traverse from the vagina, through the uterus, and into the fallopian tube to fertilize the egg.

Clomiphene citrate: An oral medication commonly used to stimulate ovulation in women by promoting the release of hormones that stimulate follicle growth.

Congenital adrenal hyperplasia (CAH): An abnormal condition where the adrenal gland produces too much androgen due to an enzyme deficiency. It often leads to hirsutism in the female.

Corpus luteum: A temporary endocrine structure that forms in the ovary after ovulation. It produces progesterone, which is essential for maintaining early pregnancy.

Cryopreservation: The process of freezing and storing biological materials (i.e., sperm, eggs, embryos) at very low temperatures for future use.

Cyst: A fluid-filled sac that can develop in an ovary or other parts of the reproductive system.

Dilation and curettage (D&C): A surgical procedure to remove tissue from inside the uterus, often performed after a miscarriage or for diagnostic purposes.

Dominant genetic disease: A disease characterized by the presence of a single, abnormal gene. Since 50% of children inherit the genetic condition, the gene can be screened in the embryo using PGT-M.

Donor egg: An egg provided by a healthy woman (donor) to be fertilized and transferred to another woman (recipient or intended parent).

Donor sperm: Sperm provided by a healthy man (donor) for use in fertility treatments.

Ectopic pregnancy: A pregnancy that implants outside the uterus, most commonly in the fallopian tube, which is not viable and can be life-threatening.

Egg retrieval (also called transvaginal oocyte retrieval): A procedure in IVF where mature eggs are collected from the ovaries using a needle guided by ultrasound. Also known as oocyte retrieval.

Embryo: A fertilized egg that has begun to divide and develop.

Embryo transfer (ET): The procedure in IVF where one or more embryos are placed into the uterine cavity. There are two main forms.

Endometrial biopsy (EMBx): The process where a small flexible catheter is inserted into the uterine cavity and a sample of the endometrium is taken. Often used to look for evidence of a low-grade infection.

Endometrial receptivity array (ERA): A diagnostic test that assesses the optimal time for embryo transfer by analyzing gene expression in the endometrial lining. While not thought to be useful in the preparation of the first ET, it may provide important information in cases of embryo transfer failures.

Endometriosis: A condition in which tissue similar to the lining of the uterus (endometrium) grows outside the uterus, often on the ovaries, fallopian tubes, or other pelvic organs, leading to pain and infertility.

Endometrium: The inner lining of the uterus where an embryo implants and grows. It sheds (menses) roughly two weeks after ovulation if no implantation occurs.

Estradiol: An estrogen hormone primarily produced by the follicles in the ovary. Rising levels indicate a maturing egg.

Fallopian tubes: Two thin tubes that extend from the uterus to the ovaries, providing a passageway for eggs to travel from the ovaries to the uterus and where fertilization typically occurs.

Fellowship: An intense three-year training program following an obstetrics and gynecology residency to focus on the care of reproductive endocrinology and infertility patients.

Fertile window: The time during a woman's cycle when ejaculated sperm into the vagina is able to enter the cervical mucous and move into the fallopian tube to fertilize the egg. It starts roughly three days before ovulation and ends the day after ovulation. The OPK test will predict when a woman is in her fertile window, indicating time for intercourse to attempt pregnancy.

Fertilization: The fusion of a sperm and an egg to form a zygote. In IVF, it is detected the day after insemination or ICSI by the presence of two pronuclei (one egg, one sperm).

Fibroids (uterine): Non-cancerous growths that develop in the wall or cavity of the uterus, which can sometimes interfere with fertility or pregnancy.

Follicle: A fluid-filled sac in the ovary containing an immature egg (oocyte).

Follicle-stimulating hormone (FSH): A hormone produced by the pituitary gland that stimulates the growth and development of follicles in the ovaries and sperm production in men. A persistently high level above 40 IU/L indicates menopause.

Follicular phase: The first part of the menstrual cycle during which follicles mature in the ovaries. The release of the dominant follicle begins the second phase of the cycle, called the luteal phase.

Fresh ET: A blastocyst is transferred into the uterus five days after the egg retrieval. This is not used when genetic testing is done, or the level of progesterone or estradiol gets too high before the trigger shot.

Frozen ET (FET): After a blastocyst is frozen, the uterus is carefully prepared to receive the thawed blastocyst, usually on the sixth day of progesterone preparation of the endometrium.

Gamete: A reproductive cell (sperm in males, egg in females).

Gamete intrafallopian transfer (GIFT): A surgical procedure where an egg and thousands of sperm are placed into the distal end of the fallopian tube. Rarely used today, it was more common in the 1980s and 1990s when IVF success rates were low.

Genetic counselor (GC): An induvial who possesses training and expertise in the field of human genetics.

Gestational carrier: A woman who carries a pregnancy for another person or couple, with no genetic connection to the baby.

Gonadotropins: Hormones (FSH and LH) that stimulate the gonads (ovaries and testes) to produce sex hormones and gametes. Often used as injectable medications in fertility treatment.

Granulosa cells: The cells of the ovary that surround the developing and mature egg. The cumulus complex are those granulosa cells that are in the closest proximity to the egg. During the egg retrieval, many granulosa cells are also removed.

Hirsutism: An abnormal condition where a woman has too much hair growth, typically on her face or abdomen, often caused by the overproduction of androgens by either the ovary or the adrenal gland.

Hormone replacement therapy (HRT): Medications containing hormones to replace those that the body no longer produces, often used to prepare the uterus for embryo transfer in frozen embryo cycles.

Human chorionic gonadotropin (hCG) trigger shot: An injection of hCG given to trigger the final maturation of eggs and induce ovulation, typically 36 hours before egg retrieval.

Hydrosalpinx: A condition where a fallopian tube is blocked and filled with fluid, which can negatively impact fertility.

Hypothalamic amenorrhea (HA): A condition in women leading to anovulation. It is characterized by low levels of FSH and LH, often caused by factors that inhibit the release of gonadotropin releasing hormone (GnRH) from the hypothalamus. Common conditions that lead to HA are exercise, eating disorders, stress, and low body fat.

Hypothalamus: The area of the brain just superior to the pituitary. It sends signals to the pituitary, causing release of many important hormones involved in daily living such as FSH, LH, TSH, ACTH, growth hormone, oxytocin, anti-diuretic hormone, and prolactin.

Hysterectomy: The surgical removal of the uterus, including the fundus and the cervix.

Hysterosalpingogram (HSG): An X-ray procedure used to evaluate the patency of the fallopian tubes and the shape of the uterus.

Hysteroscopy: A procedure in which a thin, lighted telescope (hysteroscope) is inserted into the uterus through the cervix to visualize the uterine cavity. Polyps, fibroids, and scar tissue in the uterine cavity can often be removed during hysteroscopy.

Implantation: The process by which an embryo attaches to the inner lining of the uterus (endometrium). This typically occurs roughly seven days after ovulation once the blastocyst hatches out of the zona pellucida.

Infertility: The inability to conceive after a certain period of regular unprotected intercourse (typically one year for women under 35, six months for women 35 and older). The definition has expanded to also include women who need the services of an infertility clinic to conceive, such as single women or those involved in a same-sex relationship.

Intracytoplasmic sperm injection (ICSI): A specialized IVF procedure in which a single sperm is injected directly into an egg to facilitate fertilization. Often used in cases of male factor infertility.

Intrauterine insemination (IUI): A fertility treatment where prepared sperm are placed directly into the uterus around the time of ovulation.

In vitro fertilization (IVF): A process of fertilization where an egg is combined with sperm outside the body (in vitro) in a laboratory dish.

Irregular Periods: Menstrual cycles that vary significantly in length, flow, or frequency, often indicating hormonal imbalances or ovulatory dysfunction.

Karyotype: The test to determine the number of chromosomes found in an individual, fetus, or embryo. Often done in cases of recurrent pregnancy loss and in IVF prior to embryo transfer.

Laparoscopy: A minimally invasive surgical procedure that involves inserting a thin, lighted instrument (laparoscope) through a small incision in the abdomen to visualize and sometimes treat pelvic organs. This is the procedure used to diagnose and treat endometriosis, pelvic scar tissue, and some types of uterine fibroids.

LH surge: A rapid increase in LH levels that precedes ovulation, often tested with an OPK test kit.

Luteal phase: The second half of the menstrual cycle, after ovulation, when the corpus luteum produces progesterone.

Luteinizing hormone (LH): A hormone produced by the pituitary gland that triggers ovulation in women and stimulates testosterone production in men.

Male factor infertility: Infertility caused by issues related to the male reproductive system, such as low sperm count, poor sperm motility, or abnormal sperm morphology.

Maternal fetal medicine (MFM): Specialists who have done a fellowship in high-risk obstetrics. They are often consulted when there is the potential for a complicated pregnancy.

Menopause: The natural cessation of menstruation and ovarian function, typically occurring around age 50. In 1% of women, it occurs before the age of 35. It is diagnosed by the presence of persistently high FSH levels.

Methotrexate (MTX): A chemotherapeutic agent that has been shown to medically treat an ectopic pregnancy if it is found early. It is given usually as a single injection with close follow-up of symptoms and hCG levels.

Morphology (sperm): The shape and structure of sperm.

Motility (sperm): The ability of sperm to move effectively.

Neosalpingostomy: A laparoscopic technique where a blocked fallopian tube (hydrosalpinx) is opened up to attempt pregnancy. Most women choose to move into IVF, but some patients try tubal surgery first. While the tube may stay open, it frequently doesn't function well and can lead to ectopic pregnancies.

Oocyte: A female egg cell.

Oophorectomy: The surgical removal of an ovary.

Ovarian hyperstimulation syndrome (OHSS): A potential complication of fertility treatments, particularly IVF, characterized by enlarged ovaries and fluid accumulation in the abdomen due to an exaggerated response to fertility medications. OHSS occurs more frequently in women with a high AMH.

Ovarian reserve: A woman's reproductive potential, indicating the number and quality of eggs remaining in her ovaries. Ovarian reserve is most frequently measured by AMH.

Ovaries: The female reproductive glands that produce eggs and female hormones (estrogen and progesterone).

Ovulation: The release of a mature egg from the ovary, roughly 36–40 hours after the initiation of the LH surge.

Ovulation predictor kit (OPK): An over-the-counter test purchased at a pharmacy that alerts the woman of an impending ovulation prior to the egg release. This is helpful to document ovulation and know that the couple is in the fertile window.

Pelvic inflammatory disease (PID): An infection of the female reproductive organs that can cause damage to the fallopian tubes and lead to infertility.

PGT for aneuploidy (PGT-A): Used to verify an accurate number of chromosomes (46) in the blastocyst, referred to as euploid. Too few or too many chromosomes is referred to as aneuploid.

PGT for monogenic diseases (PGT-M): Used to detect a specific genetic defect in the blastocyst, usually done in cases where a parent carries a dominant genetic defect or both parents carry the same recessive genetic defect.

PGT for polygenic diseases (PGT-P): Used to evaluate the chance of an embryo possessing a polygenic condition.

PGT for structural rearrangements (PGT-SR): Used to verify the correct number of chromosomes in the embryo when one of the parents carries a balanced translocation.

Pituitary gland: The "master gland" positioned at the base of the brain. It secretes hormones that affect many functions of the body, including ovulation, growth, milk production, and the thyroid.

Polycystic ovarian syndrome (PCOS): A common hormonal disorder in women characterized by irregular periods, excess androgen levels, and multiple small antral follicles in the ovaries, leading to ovulatory dysfunction and infertility.

Polyp: A non-cancerous glandular growth that can occur in many parts of the body, including the uterus. If large, they are often removed by hysteroscopy to facilitate conception.

Pregnancy of unknown location (PUL): A pregnancy that cannot be determined to reside in the uterine cavity. These are often failing uterine pregnancies that did not make a gestational sac (that can be seen on ultrasound) or an ectopic pregnancy. They must be followed carefully to avoid tubal rupture if an ectopic exists.

Preimplantation genetic testing (PGT): Specialized genetic testing done on the embryo prior to embryo transfer. There are several forms used in IVF.

Progesterone: A hormone produced primarily by the corpus luteum and placenta, essential for preparing the uterine lining for implantation and maintaining pregnancy. A small amount is also made daily by the adrenal gland.

Prolactin: A hormone that stimulates milk production. Elevated levels can interfere with ovulation.

Recessive genetic disease: A medical disease characterized by the presence of two abnormal genes, one typically from the mother and the other typically from the father. The presence of only one defective gene does not typically lead to disease.

Recurrent pregnancy loss (RPL): Defined as a woman with two to three first trimester pregnancy losses in a row with the same partner.

Reproductive endocrinologist (fertility doctor or REI): A physician specializing in the diagnosis and treatment of female reproductive disorders and infertility, who often oversees IVF cycles. Following medical school and obstetrics and gynecology residency, they undergo an intense three-year fellowship focused exclusively on reproductive endocrinology and infertility.

Reproductive psychiatrist: A psychiatrist with extra training and experience in the psychological effects of infertility.

Reproductive urologist: A urologist with extra training and experience in the treatment of male factor infertility.

Residency: An intense multi-year training following medical school to learn the practice of an area in medicine. Experts in fertility care do a residency in obstetrics and gynecology prior to their fellowship.

Saline infusion sonohysterography (SIS): A procedure done in the office where saline is infused into the uterine cavity, allowing for the diagnosis of polyps, fibroids, scar tissue, or uterine anomalies. Often the fluid can be seen traversing the fallopian tubes, thereby showing tubal patency.

Salpingectomy: The removal of a fallopian tube, often because of an ectopic pregnancy or a hydrosalpinx.

Semen analysis: A laboratory test that evaluates the quantity and quality of sperm in a semen sample.

Sperm: The male reproductive cell.

Sperm morphology: The shape and structure of sperm.

Sperm motility: The movement of sperm.

Sperm washing: A laboratory procedure to separate healthy, motile sperm from seminal fluid and other cells, used for IUI and IVF.

Stimulation (ovarian): The process of administering fertility medications to stimulate the ovaries to produce multiple follicles and eggs.

Subchorionic hematoma: A collection of blood between the uterine wall and the chorion (outer membrane of the gestational sac), which can occur in early pregnancy and lead to on-and-off bleeding during the first trimester.

Surrogacy: Another term for the process of using a gestational carrier.

Testicles: The male reproductive glands that produce sperm and testosterone.

Testosterone: The primary male sex hormone, essential for sperm production and male sexual characteristics.

Theca cells: The ovarian cells that are often adjacent to the granulosa cells. They primarily respond to LH with the production of androgens. Theca cell hyperfunction can lead to hirsutism in women.

Thyroid-stimulating hormone (TSH): A hormone produced by the pituitary gland that stimulates the thyroid gland. Abnormal thyroid function can affect fertility.

Transvaginal ultrasound: An ultrasound procedure performed with a transducer inserted into the vagina, used to visualize the uterus, ovaries, and follicles during fertility treatment.

Trigger shot: A shot given to cause final maturation of the egg(s), leading to either ovulation or egg retrieval. There are two commonly used trigger shots, namely hCG or a GnRH agonist.

Tubal anastomosis: A surgical procedure to remove the ligated portions of the fallopian tubes and put them back together, offering a chance at conception. However, due to higher success rates, most women choose to undergo IVF rather than tubal surgery.

Uterus: The hollow, muscular organ in the female pelvis where a fertilized egg implants and a fetus develops during pregnancy. It consists of both the cervix and the uterine fundus and allows transport of sperm from the vagina into the fallopian tube where fertilization occurs naturally.

Varicocele: An enlargement of veins in the scrotum, which can affect sperm production and quality in men.

Window of implantation: The time during the luteal phase when the endometrium is most receptive to the blastocyst. In most women, the endometrium is most receptive to the embryo on the sixth day of progesterone exposure.

Zona pellucida: The outer protective layer that surrounds an egg.
Zygote: A fertilized egg before it begins to divide.

CHAPTER 1

JOY COMES IN THE MORNING

When I was growing up, Christmas Eve always trumped every other day of the year. It was better than my birthday, better than a family vacation, better than the last day of school, and even better than Christmas Day. I would sleep late, stay in my pajamas all morning, and watch black-and-white movies such as *Holiday Inn* or *Christmas in Connecticut* with my older sister. The crisp Tennessee winter afternoon would entice us to go outside in the woods and climb trees, swinging on ropes from one tree to the next. Once we built a small fort by the creek, useful for imprisoning younger neighbors who wandered into our domain. Late in the afternoon, Mom would yell from the back door and beckon us home to get ready for a special church service. Christmas Eve evening was perhaps our most settled tradition of the year. For a Southern boy from a working family, getting all spiffed up in our fancy clothes was a once or twice a year occurrence, making it very special in my young eyes.

Our church was small with fewer than 50 people, so making an appearance on Christmas Eve was important. It would definitely be noticed if we skipped. After church, we would eat a meal that Mom prepared, specializing in Southern comfort food.

My dad was loved and knew everyone in town. He would spend lazy afternoons wandering the downtown, talking to buddies, and stopping by the local coffee shop and pawn shop. My mom, on the other hand, was more private. She spent most of her free time doing crossword puzzles in front of the TV or watching a soap opera or a game show. So special family times and special meals were enjoyed by my father but cherished by my mother.

On Christmas Eve, Mom usually prepared her go-to meal—meatloaf, mashed potatoes, green beans with just the right amount of lard thrown in, and those small rolls always on aisle three of the Piggly Wiggly. The finest restaurant in town or the local barbecue place called the Hut was no match for this. Our house was small with a kitchen at one end, three bedrooms at the other end, and a den sandwiched in between. There was no basement, only a tiny attic, and no garage—just a carport. The carport door opened into the kitchen, and after two small steps, you were at our tiny dining table. You could almost stand in the center of our kitchen and touch every counter. On Christmas Eve, we would sit down at our small table and do something my parents did not really like to do—turn off *I Love Lucy* while we ate.

After dinner, sticking with tradition, Floyd and Bertha would come over. They never had children and counted me as their son. Most of those in our small town assumed Bertha was my grandmother, the woman who loved me above all others. I loved her deeply. So, there it was—watching movies, playing in the woods, getting all spiffed up, going to church in my best clothes, and having Bertha come for a visit. It was a perfect day that filled a young Southern boy's heart with absolute contentment.

In addition, just when you might think Christmas Eve could not get any better, my family opened our gifts. After Mom's special meal and an extra helping of banana pudding made from scratch, we sat around our aluminum tree, mesmerized by the pinwheel shining red, blue, green, and yellow lights on the tree, and opened gifts, all the while cherishing this special family time. I would never dream of missing a Christmas Eve at my house.

So Christmas Eve had always been a special time for me—until that night.

I completed medical school at Vanderbilt University in Nashville, staying in my home state where I felt most comfortable. Then came time for me to start my four-year obstetrics and gynecology training. I was married during medical school, and after graduation we decided to move from Tennessee to Connecticut to start my residency. I was in a very vulnerable stage of life. We knew no one in Connecticut. We had never lived outside of Tennessee, so Connecticut seemed like a foreign land.

I was six months into my residency, long enough to be exhausted yet not long enough to see the light at the end of the tunnel. Working at least 100 hours a week and never seeing my young wife, I thought life was terrible. And just when I thought it couldn't get any worse, I was on call in obstetrics on Christmas

Eve, my favorite day. As an intern, I had no leverage. I did what I was told and went where I was sent. Not only was I far from my family over the holidays but I had to work on Christmas Eve and into Christmas morning. My wife was a great comfort to me during my residency in Connecticut, but all other family members and my closest friends were a thousand miles away. How could this be Christmas?

My night on call was terrible. Being the on-call physician meant no or very little sleep. Even though I only had six months under my belt, I was the only doctor in the busy, Hartford hospital. In addition to being very sad and somewhat angry, I was also a bit scared. But they always assigned a senior-level resident as backup in case I needed help. It was a badge of honor to handle everything on my own, so I was persevering between deliveries and the ER so I wouldn't have to bother the senior resident. I wore that badge proudly yet with reluctance on this terrible night.

My backup resident was Steve, perhaps my favorite coworker. He was kind, a good teacher, and a great chief resident. He was tall with black curly hair and a commanding presence. Steve was raised Jewish in the Northeast, so on the surface, he and I had little in common. Yet on this particular night, we had everything in common as co-residents trying to survive obstetrics and gynecology training—everything except he was home with his family, not spending a stressful and lonely night in the hospital. Steve could not have known the depth of my despair. But he must have had an inkling, because at 9:00 p.m. on Christmas Eve, he appeared in the delivery suite, grabbed my hand, and said, "Come with me."

Steve took me down the hall and around the corner to the department's administrative offices. I thought, *What is going on? Are they firing me?* We entered the first office where the secretary typically sat during the day. Steve then took out a key and opened the large wooden door in the corner, the special door into the hospital chairperson's office. As a young and vulnerable intern, fear was running through my mind. He took my hand and guided me into the chairperson's seat, a large, executive, leather chair. Wow! This was hallowed ground. On the right side of the desk was an old black phone with a rotary dial. I still had no idea why Steve had left his home on Christmas Eve and brought me into this plush office.

Then Steve did something that touched me at a very deep level. He said, "Give me your beeper. I will be the intern for a while. This phone can call anywhere in the world. Make as many phone calls as you wish." Then he was gone in a flash.

In the days before cell phones and free long-distance calling, being relieved of my beeper was quite a gift.

I was stunned. To this day, words fail me when trying to express my gratitude to Steve. Sitting there that night, however, I did not waste any time pondering why. I still cannot remember how many phone calls I made, but I called almost everyone I knew. That one act of kindness did so much to help me cope during a very difficult time in my life. After a while, my sense of duty caught up to me, and I left the office to find Steve. He probably does not know to this day how necessary he was to me on that most precious and most miserable of nights.

As I took my beeper back, I got a page from the delivery suite. According to Carmen, the nurse, there was a woman in labor getting ready to deliver. She had no attending physician, so I was it. But it took a strange turn for me. Carmen said, "She is placing her baby for adoption and doesn't want to see it." Obstetrics should be fun and happy. *You're asking me to catch the baby and hand it off to the pediatrician, never allowing the mom to see it? Really?*

Carmen was a special nurse. She was wiser than her years, a dynamo who was constantly moving. Her hair, a dominant feature atop her 5-foot, 100-pound frame, was jet black and peppered with white. Before my internship started, the more senior residents explained that Carmen would take care of me. She loved residents and took it upon herself to be their mother. She didn't have to take on that burden. She could easily have settled into a nice life doing her job and minding her own business. And she was superb at her job. When Carmen gave us advice, we followed it. Period. It was an odd relationship because as a doctor, I was in authority over Carmen. Authority is often positional, granted because of a title such as president, CEO, or captain. But the more powerful authority is forged through trial and error, through experience, from learning and growing through mistakes. I might have been granted the title, but Carmen held the real authority. I was smart enough to follow her direction because I felt it would make me a better doctor and help me survive this most difficult year. We both loved this strange relationship—a kid with a title but no experience taking direction from an Italian "mother" who knew how to take care of her "children."

The delivery itself was uneventful, and the room was sullen. The young woman pushed like a pro but cried the whole time.

I think I did too. As I clamped the cord and bundled the baby up in a blanket, hiding her from the mother, I was struck by the immense love just witnessed by all in the room. How can someone love so unconditionally? How can you nurture a baby for nine months, feel every kick and movement, and then hand it over to another mother, never to get a "thank you, Mom"? How can a mother so young, so inexperienced, make such a selfless gesture? First there was Steve's incredible generosity and now this mother's self-sacrifice. To me, this night came to symbolize unconditional love, the kind of love that allows a person to become who they are called to be, the kind of love I experienced as a child, longed to give a future child, and witnessed in the darkest despair of this young woman's life. Such love is a force, the only force that can change the world.

I finished my job, making sure the woman was okay. Later that night, before the dawn of day, I got a call from Carmen. She told me to discharge the woman. "Already?" I asked. But this was Carmen, the one who taught me so much. She taught me during this terrible ordeal that medical guidelines are only guidelines and not rules. This young woman needed to get home to her family and close this chapter of her life. However, it did not seem right to me. I wanted to talk more with her, perhaps even discuss whether she should try to raise this child. I didn't understand this love, so selfless. I wanted her to embrace the child and love her through childhood, school, those awful first dates, and into college. But I was wrong. She had already performed the greatest act of selfless love and didn't need all those things I thought she needed.

Maturity is not simply a function of age. Wisdom, while perhaps a gift, is often forged through trials. Adversity has a way of focusing our spirit and mind so the important things in life become evident. It's not that the superficial experiences that make up the better part of our day are unimportant. Those random and spontaneous acts are often what make life interesting and give it spice. But when adversity comes and despair hits you in the face, pay attention. It may be a time where you can strip off all the clutter and focus, allowing some wisdom to creep in.

I was lucky and got to sleep for about an hour. I woke up around 8:00 a.m. and looked out my window to see a light snowfall amidst a sunrise. It was a beautiful sight. As I looked down at the entrance to the hospital, I noticed a young couple embracing their new child, the one I had delivered. The man was tall and thin, dressed in a black overcoat. The woman was struggling to find the right way to hold a child, having never done it and yet knowing that she could not hand it back.

The man's hand rested on the woman's shoulder as he looked on the scene from his height, about a foot above his wife and new daughter. While I was too far away to see, I am sure there were tears in their eyes. They arrived at the hospital, broken by their infertility and despair, but left a mom and a dad full of hope for their future. I felt the many facets of the previous night's unconditional love.

The young pregnant woman's character, while still forming, changed for the better that lonely Christmas Eve. A deposit was made into her soul that could not be withdrawn. She maintained her dignity in the depths of her despair. While we did not have a deep conversation, I felt she believed in herself and knew that

28

grief would eventually pass. Life has a way of sometimes bringing joy after a time of grief. I wanted this joy to come not only to her but also to a lonely couple whose life would never be the same. A young doctor whose character was in the process of forming was also forever changed by her sacrifice. I wonder if the adopting couple ever called her. Justice would demand a thank you call. But I believe the young woman never wanted or expected it. Unconditional love does not need a thank you call.

I was hooked. While I had considered specializing in fertility treatments, I now knew my career path. I wanted the privilege of walking with someone through the valley of despair as well as the pinnacle of satisfaction. My awful, terrible, no-good Christmas Eve in the moment of a tearful delivery and two acts of unconditional love turned into one of my best Christmas Eves ever.

Joy does come in the morning.

Dr. Deaton's Prescription: Even when things do not go your way, love has a way of taking you to a better place. Love that you give unconditionally does not demand a response. Love should be received as it is given—imperfect, tarnished by the world, but given freely from an honest heart who is, like you, learning to love. My prescription for you is to give love recklessly and receive love gratefully.

How will you follow this prescription?

FINDING STRENGTH AMIDST YOUR INFERTILITY

Embarking on the path of trying to build a family can be profoundly challenging, often stirring emotions you never anticipated. It's a journey that can feel deeply personal and, at times, overwhelmingly difficult. Yet even as you navigate these turbulent waters, please hold onto this truth: *You will find your way through this.* Whether your path leads to the children you long for or takes an unexpected turn in creating your family, the intense pain of this season in your life will eventually recede.

Furthermore, difficult times often forge resilience and deepen our understanding of ourselves and our relationships. Allow yourself moments of introspection. What are you learning about your inner strength? How are your connections with others evolving? The insights gained during this period can become an indelible part of who you are.

Having witnessed the complexities of this journey for many years, I've come to understand some fundamental truths. First, infertility does not define you. It is not your identity but rather a significant challenge you are facing and one that will pass.

Second, the feeling of not measuring up (often referred to as shame) can be a heavy burden. Many experiencing infertility grapple with a sense of inadequacy. Let me be clear. Your worth is inherent and unwavering, regardless of whether or not you have children. If motherhood becomes part of your story, your children will enrich it, but your value and your unique essence exist independently.

Third, the journey of infertility can be profoundly isolating, often fueled by feelings of shame. When we feel we are falling short, our natural instinct is to withdraw. That can lead to avoiding social gatherings, places of worship, interactions with pregnant friends, and even cherished family events. This isolation can create a deep sense of loneliness. I urge you to resist complete withdrawal. While sharing your struggles with everyone may not be the right approach, be sure to identify one or two trusted individuals—perhaps a close friend or partner—you can be completely open with about your feelings and emotions. Their support can be invaluable. Try not to avoid all social engagements. Seek out those who bring you comfort and strength. If faced with questions about children, it will suffice to give a gentle response such as "We're still figuring out the timing." It is perfectly acceptable to decline events that you know will be emotionally draining and particularly difficult for you such as celebrations heavily focused on children.

Fourth, don't let infertility put your life on hold. I've heard countless individuals and couples say, "We can't plan that trip in case we get pregnant" or "I can't pursue that promotion because of potential treatment." Continue to live your life fully in the midst of this journey. Postponed dreams and lost hope can erode your joy. Don't allow that to happen.

Finally, the emotional landscape of infertility is often described as a roller coaster, and that analogy rings true. There will be highs and lows—the joy of a positive test followed by devastating news of an imminent miscarriage, the anticipation of a treatment cycle met with delays, the initial hope of many fertilized eggs that ultimately don't develop into embryos. During these inevitable ups and downs, lean on your support system, whether it's your partner, a close friend, or a counselor. Do not navigate this emotional terrain in isolation. Share what you are feeling. And always remember that this roller coaster will eventually come to a stop. Seek out moments of growth and connection along the way and allow compassionate souls to offer you comfort and support.

CHAPTER 2

SEVEN EMBRYOS, TWO COUPLES, AND A NURSE

It was several years ago, and I was sitting at my desk having a cup of coffee, not really wanting to get anything done and definitely not wanting to think too hard about work. Angela, my faithful nurse and IVF coordinator of many years, walked in with a hopeful look in her eyes—you know, the kind of look that can lead to trouble. Before I could say good morning, she said, "Our couple, the Tuckers, have five frozen embryos and can't decide what to do with them. They tried to donate them anonymously to an organization but weren't comfortable with their office. They would like for us to find a couple to adopt them." So far, this sounded great. I love embryo donation. Many couples who cannot have biological offspring would love to adopt embryos. In addition to blessing a couple, this experience also gives embryos a chance to develop into a child.

Then Angela said, "But they would like to get to know the couple and approve them before any decision is made." On the surface, this request seemed very reasonable and logical, but at its core was a complexity that caused me incredible anxiety.

"Are you crazy?!" came out of my mouth before I could even think. Within seconds, all the ethical and legal issues flooded through my mind. What if they do not like the couple we choose? Are we willing to convince a couple who has tried IVF without success and resolved themselves to their infertility and moved on with their life to come back and try again? What if this time the Tuckers' embryos don't work? What if the Tuckers change their mind after the birth and want their biological kids back? What if . . . what if . . . what if? The potential disasters were too numerous to process in those minutes before my day was to begin, in those precious moments while I tried to enjoy a cup of coffee.

Perhaps a bit of history would be helpful here. The Tuckers were a delightful couple who went through IVF and had a successful outcome with the birth of a beautiful daughter, Grace. The mother, Jessica Tucker, then returned for a second attempt and had another success following her first frozen embryo transfer. A healthy young boy, Pierce, emerged nine months later, and their family was now complete. But here's the problem. They still had five frozen embryos in storage. Following their second child, a local organization approached them to discuss the ethics of embryo freezing and their plans for their frozen embryos. Most couples use their frozen embryos for more children, but roughly 15% decide to either discard the embryos or donate them to another couple, usually anonymously. The Tuckers had mixed feelings, or perhaps they were in disagreement.

They did not want more children, and yet they wanted to give their embryos a chance. However, they were not comfortable with anonymous embryo donation, never knowing the fate of "their" children. Occasional updates or yearly pictures were not enough. They wanted more involvement, which brings me to the current dilemma. I understood their position. I love it when a couple has completed their family, has embryos in storage, and then decides to donate the remaining embryos. I also wish to give all embryos a chance.

These frozen embryos were created for the Tuckers and were genetically and emotionally linked to them. I understood their desire to give them a chance. I understood the Tuckers' longing to be part of their lives. I understood that they did not want to give birth to any more children themselves. All my training and every rational thought in my mind was saying, "Just say no." My mind was saying, "Just donate the embryos anonymously." But my heart was saying something else.

For a medical professional, the legal and ethical traps of known embryo donation are daunting. The Tuckers as the genetic parents wanted to be involved in the children's lives, but legally, who would get to make the important decisions? Does genetic continuity with a child give the parent a unique decision-making perspective that is superior to the parents who actually take care of the child? As the years pass, would the child be drawn to the genetic parents, leaving the parents who had sacrificed all those years in heartache? While I realize that genes are very important, do they define the parent-child relationship? Would the genetic parent feel an entitlement that is not supported by the parents who actually did the hard work?

As a fertility physician, I had witnessed countless sacrifices by people longing to be parents. As a parent, I was also personally aware of some of those sacrifices. I didn't want years of pain negated by a genetic parent whose only parental claim was genetic. Are genes actually that important? Which parent would the courts support in a contest between the adults? I was conflicted, and all these questions and more came flooding into my mind.

Angela was still standing in the doorway, smiling a somewhat devious smile. She was a fantastic nurse, a caring individual, and a woman who was accustomed to getting her way. I hired her while I was working at Wake Forest to be the IVF nurse coordinator and then announced a few months later that I was leaving. Fortunately, she chose to follow me to a new program. She had the ability to pour herself into the details of an IVF cycle while at the same time nurturing and overseeing the big-picture aspects of the program. She enjoyed authority and saw herself as a leader. Before Angela, I had hired several IVF coordinators. Some had lasted one day (really), and three other fantastic IVF coordinators had each been with me for four years. I was fortunate.

Amazingly, Angela had held the job for 10 years. She had enough self-confidence to handle stress and failure. The emotions of IVF never really seemed to get to her. There was something special about her. And on this particular day, I instinctively knew who was in charge.

I relented to Angela, as I often did. I understood the conflict too well. I said to Angela, "How are we going to match them to the right couple?" It was at that moment that I learned I was a mere spectator in this grand design, forfeiting all authority to the collective scheming of my office.

"Oh," said Angela, "we've already found the perfect couple, and the entire office agrees." The plot appeared before my eyes, just when I thought I was in charge.

Roughly one year earlier, our office said our goodbyes to a wonderful couple who had exhausted all means of having a child. It was a tender goodbye since the office loved them so much. She had poor egg quality and had failed IVF. That was the end of the road as far as they were concerned. They chose to accept their family as it was—husband and wife—that is, until Jessica and Angela came up with their idea. In fact, I also discovered that Jessica had come by the office earlier and learned from Angela of a wonderful couple who left the practice after exhausting all their options. Everyone, including Jessica, wanted to help them.

The office arranged a meeting between the two couples. Going into that meeting, I was very nervous but had to concentrate on an office full of patients. I'm sure the women I had to see that day noticed that I was a bit distracted. All the disastrous scenarios played out in my mind that day. In the end, not one of my fears came to be. The meeting between the couples was a huge success. Not only did they agree to proceed, but they also became friends.

It was as if I had lost all control, yet I did not mind at all. I kept waiting for something or someone to stop the process. Surely the Tuckers would change their minds. Surely someone would back out. Surely the infatuation the four people felt for each other would die off. However, all went wonderfully. Before you knew it, I transferred two normal embryos into a new and receptive uterus. And the woman became pregnant—with twins. A couple who had given up all hope were now holding a healthy girl and a healthy boy. Now there was no going back.

These two families were uniquely linked in a way perhaps no two other families are. Situations sometimes occur that forever link two families. Families often share joy as in the marriage of their two children. Some families share grief when their children suffer a common tragedy. But these two couples were now linked in a very unique and deep way, all perhaps equally embracing the role of parents in all the children's lives. We can easily see one or two parents, but four is much more difficult to imagine.

To witness a couple raising their own biological children while at the same time watching another couple raise two more of their biological children—wow! Would they tell the children? Who is the mom, or are there two moms? Would the children figure it out on their own? Would the two families fight over how to parent the twins? Would the Tuckers be blamed for the twins' lot in life? There were so many questions for what might lie ahead, but there was also so much love and respect between these two couples. Would they embrace this linkage fully and co-parent, or would they keep a separation between the families? How would they navigate keeping the kids from dating each other?

While I support the fact that couples get to decide what happens to their unwanted embryos, I celebrate when they decide to give them a fighting chance. So many infertile couples want to adopt embryos, and so many embryos are no longer needed or wanted. Why not give them a chance while fulfilling a longing deep inside another couple? When the Tuckers decided to place their embryos with another couple, everyone won. One couple was not forced to have more children against their will, another couple had the greatest desire of their hearts fulfilled, and the embryos—regardless of anyone's beliefs—were given a chance. Pro-life or pro-choice did not matter.

We often need help in the course of life. In my experience, help often comes at the most unlikely time from the most unlikely person. Who would have ever dreamed that this infertile couple would need some help in allowing their embryos a chance, thereby conceding the parenting of these children to another couple? Who would have dreamed that another infertile couple, content with a decision to live without children, would be willing to bare themselves once again and step back into the emotional roller coaster of infertility care? The Tuckers were brave enough to be upfront about their issues, seek help, and open their hearts to another couple who courageously stepped into the ring again to go one more round against infertility. There was no way to predict the outcome, yet everyone moved forward with trust and expectancy.

If you are facing something tough, don't despair. Let some skilled and trusted people you know in, and you might be surprised at the help that is just on the horizon. Begin to believe and expect that there are people out there who are able to help. Reach deep down inside and summon the inner strength to find those people; they might just love to lock arms with you.

There were now several children, all genetic siblings, raised by two separate couples, one of which represented all the children's genetic parents. Both couples are friends, and all children will be raised as friends, perhaps one day to learn the truth. It's hard to even understand all the ramifications, all the ethics, and all the interesting conversations that will occur. But I'm glad there are people like these two couples in North Carolina.

And yes, if you did the math, there are three remaining embryos. This unique little village might grow over the next few years. Sometimes it does take a village.

Dr. Deaton's Prescription: We often live life in the gray zones. While it is easy when issues are black and white, we all know there are mysteries in life we must embrace. When embracing a mystery, let others in on the journey. Life is not just smooth sailing; it is also a roller coaster ride. Bring someone along with you. It is much more fun to scream with someone when life feels out of control.

My prescription for you is this. Consider the hardest thing you are facing right now and find someone to share it with. Then accept the love and help they want to give to you. Don't live life by yourself; let others in on the ride.

How will you follow this prescription?

NAVIGATING THE PATH TO PARENTHOOD: KNOWING WHEN, WHERE, AND HOW TO SEEK HELP

The traditional definition of infertility is one year of unprotected intercourse without conception. Infertility is a common unseen medical condition shared by many. In fact, infertility affects a significant portion of the population—approximately one in seven women under the age of 35, rising to one in four between 35 and 39, and reaching one in three for women over 39.

However, this standard definition doesn't fit every situation. For same-sex couples, those in long-distance relationships, or individuals with known factors that impact fertility, waiting a year would be unnecessary. Similarly, if there's a clear reason for infertility such as a prior vasectomy or early menopause, delaying action serves no purpose. While the traditional guideline might be relevant for some, it overlooks the diverse circumstances individuals and couples face.

So, when is the right time to seek help? Consider these parameters as you navigate your journey, and do not wait a year in the following situations.

- **When a year of trying naturally doesn't align with your circumstances.** This category includes same-sex couples, single individuals, couples living apart, those with frequent travel preventing timed intercourse around ovulation, and those experiencing sexual dysfunction (painful intercourse or erectile difficulties).

- **When there's a known factor affecting fertility.** Some examples are irregular menstrual cycles, prior tubal ligation or vasectomy, history of tubal pregnancies or pelvic surgery, or early menopause resulting from natural causes or medical treatments such as chemotherapy. If you face a medical crisis such as the need for aggressive chemotherapy, that could lead to early menopause.

- **If you are older and want a large family.** Remember that if you get pregnant, your next attempt might be two to three years away if you choose to breastfeed. If you are older and wait a few years for your next pregnancy, you might age out of having another child.

- **If you are over 35 and have been trying for six months.** Given the impact of age on female fertility, a shorter time frame for seeking help is recommended for those over 35.

If you are anxious about your fertility for any reason, it never hurts to seek an opinion to either begin a workup and treatment or perhaps to simply put your mind at ease.

As you might imagine, the above categories encompass a lot of women and couples. However, it is fine to wait a year if you are under 35, have regular cycles, have a straightforward gynecological history—no prior reproductive surgeries or sexually transmitted infections (STIs), — and are not worried about your future fertility. Roughly 85% of younger couples will spontaneously conceive during the first year, and time is often all that is needed.

Where Can You Find the Support You Need?

Once you've decided to seek help, where do you turn? A logical first step is often your gynecologist who can order initial tests and may suggest basic interventions such as oral fertility medications. However, it's important to be aware of certain limitations of your gynecologist's office.

- Their office may not be specifically equipped for infertility patients, potentially lacking dedicated nursing support.
- The presence of many obstetrical patients in the waiting room can be emotionally challenging for those struggling to conceive.
- The intricacies of infertility, including insurance coverage and medication authorizations, might not be their primary focus.
- Due to their broader practice, the process of obtaining tests or treatments might take longer.

So if you are older, feel particularly anxious about your fertility, or do not have an established gynecologist, you should bypass this initial step and consult an expert directly. In fact, many couples start with the expert since they don't want to waste any time.

Who are the fertility experts? They are physicians who have completed a four-year residency in obstetrics and gynecology, followed by an intensive three-year fellowship in reproductive endocrinology and infertility. Officially known as Reproductive Endocrinologists, they are commonly referred to as fertility doctors or fertility specialists. These doctors dedicate their practice to helping individuals and couples achieve pregnancy, often working within academic departments or private practices located in larger cities.

A referral is often not required to see a fertility doctor, and you are generally welcome to schedule an appointment directly. Their offices are specifically designed for fertility care, which can streamline the diagnostic and treatment process. To locate a specialist, you can ask for recommendations from friends or consult the website of the Society for Assisted Reproductive Technology (SART) at www.sart.org. The site allows you to search by geographic area and even provides data on in vitro fertilization (IVF) success rates.

Choosing the right path is a crucial early step. May you have the very best fertility team for your journey.

CHAPTER 3

ALL I EVER WANTED WAS TO BE A DAD

The embryo transfer was fairly easy. The patient had delivered two previous children, so I had no difficulty navigating the cervical canal and placing two healthy blastocysts into her uterine cavity. Each blastocyst is strong with a roughly 55% chance of implanting in the uterus. It was so quick and easy that it almost felt anticlimactic, yet I knew it might become a watershed moment for the couple. After writing a note in the chart, I went to the waiting room to tell Andy, the potential father, how the procedure went. He had decided to wait rather than be in the room with the mother. While he understood his importance in this process, he also knew that he was perceived as more of a bystander in this most important of moments. Andy wanted a voice and yet was often seen as the quiet one. When asked to sign a consent, write a check, or have blood drawn, he did his duty—quietly. His eyes were expressive, and he didn't hide his feelings. So when he was the quiet one in the room and a bit sad, I knew he wanted more.

Just after I finished describing the ease of the transfer and the high quality of the blastocysts, he said something that pierced my heart.

"All I've ever wanted was to be a dad."

I was so proud of him at that moment. Many men feel this way, and in my office, most men experience the joys of fatherhood for the first time. Most of our couples are without children, so many men come to my office very stoic, trying to be the strong one for their partner. They approach and handle infertility very differently than women. Emotions flow from the women in my office. Men, while very emotional at their core, often hold back in that tender moment as they sit next to their partners. However, if you get them alone and say the right words, emotions will flow. They are devastated over their infertility and despise the way their most important relationship has become soured. They are often in love with their wives, and yet the dream of and love for a child has replaced their partner's first love.

The desire to be a father is strong, perhaps as strong as the desire to be a mother. Yet it is often under the surface, not fully expressed. The intense emotions get in the way. They need to be strong for their partners and say, "Everything will be okay. We'll get through this together." But the loss of this dream, to be a father, often leads them into isolation, chasing other dreams that seem important to men—dreams that are often more validated by society. They seem fine climbing the corporate ladder or excelling in the world of sports, but inwardly, they are wounded and hurt.

This couple was no ordinary couple. They moved to our area needing both an egg donor and a surrogate to carry their pregnancy. They quickly found the right surrogate, and the surrogate had located a perfect egg donor, her best friend. The stage was set. Egg donation and surrogacy is a very long and frustrating process. Synchronizing the egg donor to the surrogate's uterus, making sure the day of fertilization is timed to the preparedness of the surrogate uterus, is not too challenging for my office. All the legal and governmental requirements mandated by the FDA are overwhelming. The egg donor lived in another city, so all the blood and urine testing on both women had to be coordinated between two cities. And the psychological and legal work had to be duplicated between the two women. To make it worse, roadblocks kept arising. Many couples would have given up, but this couple persevered. This one treatment cycle involved a couple, two women, several lawyers, FDA regulations, and different cities. We could feel the complexity.

Finally, it all fell into place, and we started the surrogate on hormones and the egg donor on fertility injections. The couple waited patiently, almost as spectators in this most important drama in their lives. Multiple eggs were retrieved and fertilized, and six healthy embryos developed. The surrogate was ready, and two embryos were placed into her uterus while the remaining four were frozen for later use. She understood the risk of twins but wanted to fulfill the couple's wishes. While seemingly distanced observers, the couple was well aware of their role in the process and the important impact of their decisions. During all the procedures, they had to wait patiently in the lobby.

"All I've ever wanted was to be a dad."

You see, they were a same-sex couple, two men who wanted a family but in a relationship that might never land them on a path to fatherhood. "All I ever wanted was to be a dad." I can only imagine the grief Andy must have felt early in his adult life when he realized his dream might never come true. His partner was the focused one, the one who was detail oriented. I believe at some point his dream of being a father emerged, and his partner said something like, "Don't worry. We can do this." But the many months of frustration must have been hurtful to his young soul.

Dreams are important. Without dreams, life can seem futile and pointless. Without dreams, it is easy to slip into despair or depression because life can be hard. Dreams are the secret substance of hope, and hope is the best motivator on the planet. Often our dreams are very personal, while others are based on making this world a better place. For many, both of these factors combine into several dreams. For this young man, however, his dream was extremely personal and also possibly unattainable due to his sexual orientation. Yet Andy was willing to dream something that he might never achieve. To be honest, most of us choose dreams that may be difficult but are within reach.

It takes courage to put a dream out there that may not be reached. Your dream gets people talking. It can get tiresome to keep answering questions about unanswered dreams. This predicament possibly came a little easier to this young man since he had already pursued difficult dreams. But this dream was so personal, and the loss of this dream would hurt so much. While

Andy had overcome other obstacles in his life, facing this dream head on still took courage.

The desire to be a father, a desire that is so strong, drove them to persevere against all odds. For most couples, the infertility journey is filled with obstacles, emotions, roadblocks, and failed dreams. For this couple, it was all that plus a whole lot more.

We are all unique. We all have different gifts and talents. And yet there are some common threads that unite all of humanity. Wanting to be a father, to your child or someone else, is one of those common threads. Politically, it is often hard to understand the "other side." Two gay men wanting a child may cause some to raise concerns, but those who knew these two men understood and supported their dream. In times of discord and disagreement, look for common threads that unite such as a man's desire to be a dad. The threads that unite are so much greater than the chasms that separate.

Don't be afraid to address this inward desire to be a father. While you may think you could only parent your own biological child, I doubt that is true. In my experience, men are often able to be a dad to their own children, to other children, to young men in jeopardy, or to young people who need a mentor. If you don't know how to start, find an older man and allow him to mentor you. You might feel mentally and emotionally exhausted, but you will be surprised to find how being a father brings so much energy. Give in to this dream and don't hold back. Be a dad to someone. There are a lot of young people out there who would love to have a dad.

It just may become "all you've ever wanted to be."

Dr. Deaton's Prescription: Fathering is a gift, a calling, and a lifelong challenge. Acting like a father is not gender specific. The idea of shepherding someone or something applies to all genders. We are made in a way that enables us to be fathers. If possible, dream big. Dream against all odds. Dream of ways you can be a father figure—to your own children or to those in need of a father.

Is there someone or something in your life that needs a coach or a shepherd? Do you feel drawn to be a mentor to a younger person or a fledgling organization?

Go be a mentor!

How will you follow this prescription?

A WORD OF SUPPORT FOR THE MALE PARTNER

Being the male partner in a couple experiencing infertility presents its own unique set of challenges. It's understandable that you might be grappling with a range of difficult emotions, including the following:

- **Witnessing your partner's pain:** It can be incredibly tough to see the woman you love endure the emotional toll of infertility. The feelings of loneliness, sadness, and isolation she may experience can make you feel helpless as if you've lost the connection you once shared. Many men express a deep longing to see their partner happy and whole again.

- **Dealing with the inability to "fix" it:** While men may not always express the same feelings of shame as their partners, they often struggle with the inability to resolve the situation and the potential disappointment of not becoming a father. That can lead to feelings of inadequacy, frustration, and sadness.

- **Facing the possibility of a male factor:** Discovering that sperm issues might be contributing to the difficulty in conceiving can be challenging for some men. No one wants to feel like they are preventing their partner from achieving a deeply held desire. That fear can even lead some men to avoid testing all together.

- **Navigating the impact on intimacy:** The shift from spontaneous intimacy to timed intercourse for conception can significantly alter a couple's sex life. What was once a source of pleasure can begin to feel like an obligation. Ironically, once you begin working with a fertility specialist, the pressure around timed intercourse often lessens, potentially allowing intimacy to become enjoyable again. Understanding the fertile window and having the clinic manage the timing of sperm delivery can bring a sense of relief and normalcy back to your relationship.

- **Managing the financial strain:** The cost of infertility treatment, especially without comprehensive insurance coverage, can add significant stress to a couple's lives, sometimes leading to sacrifices in other areas they enjoy such as travel or larger purchases.

So how do you navigate these complex emotions and the stress of the infertility journey? Here are some helpful tips.

Remember, it's not your fault. Even if a low sperm count is a contributing factor, it's a medical condition, just like any other. Your worth as a man is not defined by your sperm count. It's also important to understand that testosterone levels and sperm count are not directly related. High testosterone does not guarantee high sperm count, and testosterone supplementation can actually decrease sperm production to zero. So, if you're taking a testosterone derivative, let both your partner and fertility doctor know.

Trust in the effectiveness of treatment. While the process can be demanding, fertility treatments are often very successful. Remind yourself and your partner that you are likely to navigate this successfully and move forward to the next chapter of your lives.

Let intimacy be enjoyable again. Talk openly with your doctor about the impact of timed intercourse on your relationship. Trust their guidance to help alleviate the pressure and allow intimacy to return to being a source of connection and pleasure. Don't hesitate to ask any questions you have about sex and conception. Fertility specialists are accustomed to these conversations and are bound by confidentiality.

Continue living your life. Don't put your dreams and enjoyable activities on hold even though finances might be tight. Keep planning trips, pursuing hobbies, and making purchases you desire. Live your life fully while navigating infertility. While loans can add further stress, some couples are creative and speak with family members or friends to help with the financial burden.

Seek out emotional support. This journey can be emotionally taxing, and finding the right support is crucial. While many support groups and resources focus on the female experience of infertility, look for groups specifically designed for couples. The presence of other men in a group setting can often create a comfortable space for men to share their experiences and feelings. These groups may be short-term, but even a brief period of connection with other couples can be incredibly validating and open the door for deeper conversations with your partner.

Don't suffer in silence. If you can't find a suitable group, reach out to a trusted male friend, mentor, or therapist. Men are just as capable of experiencing and expressing emotions as their female partners. They often simply need the right environment and someone they feel comfortable confiding in.

Remember, you are not alone in this. Your feelings and experiences are valid. By supporting your partner and taking care of your own emotional well-being, you can navigate this journey together and emerge stronger as a couple.

CHAPTER 4

FROM ABSENCE TO ABUNDANCE

During my Vermont training, I received a page from my physician and friend, John. When I answered, he said, "Jeff, are you sitting down?" That question is not a good way for a physician to start a conversation with his patient. As you can imagine, within a few seconds, every medical catastrophe flooded my mind. Was it cancer? Did I have some rare neurological disease? Was my heart getting ready to explode?

"Amy and I are pregnant!" was his response.

"What?"

You see, John was not only my doctor and good friend, but he and Amy had been my long-time patients. They wanted a large family and had tried for many, many years without success. They came to me. Following a standard workup, I diagnosed John and Amy with longstanding unexplained infertility. In other words, even with all our science and knowledge, I couldn't tell them why they were unable to conceive. Unexplained infertility is always unsettling since patients come to doctors for answers. But it is a harsh reality of medicine that the more we learn and know, the less we understand.

For a Christian couple like John and Amy, unexplained infertility is agony. The Bible is full of references regarding the blessing of children. I can quote most of them. So a Christian couple with unexplained infertility often makes a terrible conclusion—we must be unblessed. And if I am unblessed, then either I'm doing something wrong, or God doesn't love me. While the logic might make sense, the foundation of "I am unblessed" is a lie. The conclusions built on this foundation are a lie and therefore wrong. Rather than facing infertility with some confidence, this wrong line of thinking leads many into a season of agonizing self-criticism.

Trials are very complicated. I've seen people experience trials because of bad decisions, and I've seen trials, often unwarranted, grow out of conflicts with other individuals. But perhaps more frequently, I've seen trials come out of the randomness of life. Bad things sometimes happen to good people for no reason. While it is important to understand the cause of the trial, it is more important to persevere through the trial. No storm lasts forever, and all trials pass. Having an inner fortitude to get through the storm with your self-worth intact is much more important than determining the cause of the trial. You often can't understand why an obstacle is in your path.

Fortunately, John and Amy were well-grounded and embraced the mysteries in life. Things are rarely black and white. They understood that children are a blessing but are neither the only blessing nor perhaps even the greatest blessing. They knew

God loved them, and they realized how blessed they were. Yet it still hurt, and they still wanted children. As their friend and doctor, I so wanted to help them. It hurt me too.

I really liked John and Amy. He was young (as was I), trying to establish a career in internal medicine. He had a perfect doctor demeanor—serious yet relaxed, giving medical facts and yet also able to offer wisdom about life. With curly hair and tennis shoes, it was easy to relax with him. Perhaps more important, he was able to laugh, another sign of a healthy individual. He was the kind of man I could go to for my annual physical (with all it entails) and also sit down together with a cup of coffee and discuss the multiple questions in life. I knew Amy less well but was impressed with her joy and ability to pull you into a conversation. They would make wonderful parents. To make it worse for me, John's father was also in our small community. He was very important to our integration into the town. As John and Amy struggled, I heard of it not only from them but also from John's parents. The pressure was mounting.

Unexplained infertility often leads to a long and painful journey. There are multiple office treatments that can be performed, but they only work in a minority of cases. With hope at each attempt, John and Amy went through every one of them. Fertility drugs—no success. Insemination protocols—no success. Dye study of the uterus and tubes—no success. More time and vacations—no success. We only had one option left—in vitro fertilization (IVF). Even though IVF works very well in this type of situation, it is costly and time-consuming. After many, many years of disappointment and all the fears and concerns and faith testing that go with unexplained infertility, John and Amy decided to embark on their last hope: IVF.

While this was many, many years ago, I still remember Amy's cycle. It was perfect, a reproductive endocrinologist's dream. She had a beautiful ovarian stimulation with a wonderful egg development and an easy egg retrieval. At that time, we only used light sedation. During my cases, I would often put on some music. Toward the end of the egg retrieval, I was lightly singing along to Amy Grant, feeling very full of myself. Out of nowhere, Amy said, "Jeff, is that Amy Grant singing?" A little startled, I said yes. Amy then replied, "Then let her sing!"

I'll also never forget the embryo transfer. John and a group of guys were on a trip, so Amy brought her four best friends to the transfer. We all crammed into the tiny room along with a prep cart, exam table, and several chairs, and waited for the embryos to arrive in their catheter. It was such an intimate moment shared with her four closest friends—and her gynecologist. There was a lot of laughter and chatting. The transfer was perfect, and two weeks later, I saw her positive pregnancy test come across my desk.

I yelled for my IVF nurse and wanted to celebrate. All pregnancies are special, but this one tasted especially sweet. I felt so full of life at that moment to have helped my dear friend achieve something so precious and so close to being out of his grasp. I couldn't just call John or Amy, so I did something I have never done before and never done since. I went looking for John. We worked in the same medical center, so how hard could it be? Over the course of the next hour, I went from one room to another looking for him. The medical center was very large, and I felt like a mouse in a maze, navigating hallways between buildings that don't seem to connect. At every stop, the nurse or secretary would say, "You just missed him. But I know where he is heading." And then I would go off on another journey.

Finally, I trapped him in his office and told him the incredible news. We celebrated, and then I felt a tinge of guilt over not telling Amy first. I left John alone, and he decided to give Amy the news in an exceptional way. Nine months later, they welcomed their daughter into the world. So many years of frustration and disillusionment came to a screeching halt. Their infertility was now a distant memory. This trial, which had occupied several years of their young married life, had now passed. They had endured and were now entering a new season, a little beat up perhaps but not scarred. They didn't need to understand why. They were content simply holding their daughter.

Let's go back to the phone call at the start of the story. John called me six months after their daughter was born, asked me to sit down, and said, "We're pregnant!" Amy had conceived without anyone's help (except for John's help, of course). She had conceived spontaneous twins, an uncommon event. As a fertility doctor, I know twins are not rare, but spontaneous twins occur in one out of every 100 births. So nine months later, they welcomed their two boys into the world. While this may seem like the end of the story, hold on.

Believe it or not, six months after their twins were born, John called me again, asked me to take a seat once again, and said, "We're pregnant again without any help!" Of course, my first response was, "How do you have time to have sex?" And without missing a beat, John said, "We had it once!" A few months later,

John and Amy welcomed their fourth child into the world. Two boys and two girls, all under the age of three. Who could have ever predicted this? Not in a million years.

I don't always understand why we have to face the trials that are in front of us. Why can't these trials just be removed? Why did John and Amy have to suffer all those years of infertility to end up with four children all under the age of three? While the cause may be a mystery, I do know that persevering through trials deposits something into our character that can never be removed. We grow through challenges more than during the years of plenty. I also know that we are often at our lowest point just prior to our breakthrough. The moment you're ready to give up is the moment you should fight and press through the trial to your victory.

In the ebb and flow of life, during the peaks of joy and the valleys of despair, it's easy to believe that your blessings are also coming and going. But adversities are not times when the blessings are gone. They are simply seasons of life when you can lose focus on your blessings. Consider that blessings often provide the secret ingredient that allows you to face tough situations in life. When in a valley, do you see your life as unfair and yourself as a victim? Or do you face the trial, maintain your sense of self-worth, and wait for the next blessing? You can choose to examine your life and look for burdens, or you can choose to look for the blessings that have not disappeared but simply have gone out of focus. If you're able to pay attention to the blessings, perhaps you'll see some more approaching from the distance.

Whatever you're facing, don't despair. Maintain hope, which is the motivating force behind everything you do. John often said that God was chuckling during all those years and thinking, *Just wait and be patient.* I'm so glad John and Amy persevered and moved into a land of plenty, and I'm so happy God has a sense of humor.

Dr. Deaton's Prescription: All of us will face storms and trials in our lives. Are you facing one now? In the midst of the trial, does your life seem out of control, and do you feel like a victim? Has your focus on this bad thing in your life totally drowned out all the good things in your life? Are you now focused on the trial rather than on your life?

Today, name (and perhaps even write down) some of the many blessings in your life. Think of the people who are at the heart of these blessings. Call or write one of them.

How will you follow this prescription?

THE BEAUTIFUL SYMPHONY OF THE MENSTRUAL CYCLE AND REPRODUCTION

As a reproductive endocrinologist, I am continually in awe of the elegant choreography that is the female menstrual cycle. The precise timing, hormonal synchronization, and sheer biological artistry orchestrated by a microscopic egg (roughly 120 microns in diameter) are truly remarkable. This intricate symphony unfolds in four key movements.

First, the ovary, the storehouse containing the finite number of eggs a woman will ever possess, serves as the source of all the movements.

Second, the pituitary gland, a small but mighty endocrine center at the base of the brain, conducts a cascade of crucial hormones. While often dubbed the "master gland," in the context of the menstrual cycle, it acts as the first violin, responding to the egg's lead. Its repertoire includes thyroid-stimulating hormone, growth hormone, prolactin (for lactation), oxytocin (for labor), follicle-stimulating hormone (FSH, vital for egg development), and luteinizing hormone (LH, triggering egg release or ovulation).

Third, the hypothalamus, a deeper brain region, acts as the prompter, sending signals to the pituitary. Intriguingly, the hormones produced by the developing egg influence both the pituitary and the hypothalamus, creating a delicate feedback loop.

Fourth, the uterus, the stage for potential new life, comprises three layers: the outer serosa, the muscular myometrium, and the inner endometrium. The endometrium is a particularly remarkable tissue that regenerates anew each month, defying age to provide a receptive environment for embryo implantation and sustain a pregnancy even in later reproductive years. While the eggs themselves age and may develop genetic abnormalities over time, the uterus maintains its youthful receptivity through this monthly renewal.

These four components of the female reproductive system harmonize each month with the potential to bring new life into the world. The cycle actually begins a few days before menstruation as the pituitary gland starts to release FSH. In the ovaries, two types of cells respond to FSH and LH, which are both released by the pituitary. The theca cells reside slightly away from the egg, while the granulosa cells are in direct contact with the egg. At the start of a normal menstrual cycle in a woman with a healthy egg reserve, around 30 or so antral follicles (fluid-filled sacs each containing one egg) begin to develop, all vying to become the single dominant follicle for that month. In most cycles, only one will ultimately be selected for ovulation. The LH stimulates the theca cells to produce androgens (including testosterone), which then diffuse into nearby blood vessels and the granulosa cells.

Within the granulosa cells, two critical transformations occur. First, a small percentage of these androgens are converted into estrogens through a process called aromatization. Second, this locally produced estrogen enters the bloodstream and triggers the formation of FSH receptors on the granulosa cells. That sets the stage for the competition among the approximately 30 antral follicles. The follicle with the most efficient aromatase activity will produce the most estrogen and consequently develop the highest number of FSH receptors.

As estrogen levels rise in the bloodstream (originating from all the developing antral follicles), this rising estrogen signals the pituitary to reduce its FSH output. This crucial interplay typically occurs early in the cycle before day seven (with day one being the first day of bleeding). Herein lies a beautiful principle of the cycle: As estrogen rises and FSH falls, only the antral follicle with the most FSH receptors can continue to thrive, becoming the dominant follicle. The remaining competing follicles undergo atresia, a process of programmed cell death. So, despite starting with a cohort of developing eggs, only one typically reaches maturity each month.

The next pivotal event occurs around day 12 when the estrogen level in the blood (now primarily produced by the dominant follicle) reaches a plateau of approximately 200 picograms/ml and sustains that level for about 50 hours. This sustained high estrogen level triggers the pituitary gland to release a surge of luteinizing hormone—the LH surge. This LH surge orchestrates three vital processes.

First, it initiates ovulation or the actual release of the mature egg from the ovary, which then travels into the fallopian tube. Second, it prompts the granulosa cells to shift their primary hormone production from estrogen to progesterone, thereby preparing the uterine lining (endometrium) for potential embryo implantation. That marks the beginning of the rise in progesterone levels, which will peak approximately seven days after ovulation. Third, the LH surge induces the final maturation of the egg, rendering it capable of being fertilized. Prior to the LH surge, the egg cannot be naturally fertilized.

If fertilization occurs, the resulting embryo travels down the fallopian tube and into the uterus, implanting roughly seven days after ovulation. This implantation signals the developing pregnancy to release human chorionic gonadotropin (hCG) into the bloodstream. The hCG can be measured as a positive pregnancy test. The hCG then travels to the corpus luteum (the structure that remains in the ovary after the egg is released), rescuing it from its natural decline and ensuring continued high levels of progesterone, thus preventing menstruation.

If implantation does not occur, there is no hCG signal. The corpus luteum degenerates, leading to a sharp drop in progesterone levels. This progesterone decline triggers two key events. First, it causes FSH levels to begin to rise again, initiating a new cycle even before bleeding starts. Second, it causes the uterus to shed the endometrium, resulting in menstruation. And so, the entire process begins anew with a fresh cohort of antral follicles, each vying for dominance in the next cycle—a monthly renewal that preserves the uterus's youthful receptivity.

Let's shift and discuss some relevant anatomy. The cervix—the lower, narrow end of the uterus—sits at the top of the vagina. It's the firm structure palpable during a pelvic exam and can often be felt manually by women themselves. The cervix has an opening into the vagina called the external os. This opening allows sperm to enter, but typically only when the cervical mucus is receptive during the fertile window. Unfortunately, this opening can also provide a portal for viruses and bacteria, leading to STIs. In a monogamous relationship, these infections are very uncommon.

Regarding sexual activity, the cervix is situated at the apex of the vagina in virtually all women. Regardless of sexual position, the force of male ejaculation deposits sperm onto the cervix and external os, and within seconds a small percentage of sperm navigate through the cervix and through the internal os (the opening from the cervix into the uterus). The reason men ejaculate such a large number of sperm is because only a fraction will successfully enter the cervix. Therefore, no specific sexual position has been scientifically proved to be superior for conceiving. They should all be equally effective. While some fluid and a significant portion of sperm will exit the vagina when a woman stands up, a sufficient number of sperm typically enter the cervix within moments of ejaculation. Elevating the hips after intercourse is often suggested, but it is generally not considered necessary.

Another frequent question revolves around the fertile window, the limited time each month when conception is actually possible. Women with absent or highly irregular cycles often lack a predictable fertile window and should seek medical advice to induce ovulation. In ovulatory women, the fertile window is defined by the characteristics of the cervical mucus. As estrogen levels rise in the days leading up to ovulation, the cervix produces sperm-friendly mucus. The mucus facilitates sperm transport and is typically present in sufficient quantities for only about four days per cycle. Following ovulation, progesterone levels increase, and the cervical mucus becomes thick and less permeable to sperm, effectively closing the fertile window. Combining these factors, the fertile window typically encompasses the three days preceding ovulation and the day of ovulation itself. Intercourse outside this window is unlikely to result in conception.

If timing intercourse feels like a chore, consider using an ovulation predictor kit (OPK). Starting around cycle day 10 or 11 (with day one being the first day of bleeding), these kits detect the LH surge that precedes ovulation. A positive OPK result usually indicates that ovulation will occur within the next 12 to 36 hours, making the night of the positive test firmly within the fertile window. Finally, sperm can survive in good cervical mucus for two to four days. Studies have shown that a single act of intercourse during the fertile window, such as on the day of a positive OPK, should be sufficient for conception. Therefore, abandon the notion of frequent, scheduled intercourse throughout the cycle. Focus your baby-making efforts on the day of your positive OPK and let intimacy at other times be for pleasure and connection.

CHAPTER 5

LIVING LIFE TO THE FULLEST

Experience always helps lighten someone up. I was recruited to Wake Forest for one specific purpose: to start and run a successful IVF program. As a fellow in training, I was instrumental in starting an IVF program in Vermont and helped conceive the first IVF pregnancy in the state's history. A career in IVF was very tempting to me because it afforded a niche in a cutting-edge field. It also offered me the opportunity to work with couples who are struggling with very deep emotional issues and facing some very serious ethical challenges.

When I started training in Vermont in 1987, there were only a handful of programs in the world. Due to the infancy of the field, I was also able to learn every aspect—the complex laboratory, the unique psychological insights, and the challenging medical, ethical, and legal decisions. When the program in Vermont turned successful, I knew that finding a good job would not be difficult. Winston-Salem, North Carolina, was an easy decision because it brought my family back to the South, nestled between the gorgeous Smoky Mountains and the Atlantic Ocean, to a program that wanted to excel. It was an automatic niche for me and a place my young family could call home. It was a place where springtime is magical and every day at dusk a litany of insects emerges to create a chorus of peace and tranquility.

I started my career in the summer of 1990, looking like a freshman in college. I grew a mustache so patients would stop wondering if I was really a doctor. The program was immediately blessed with the hiring of two exceptional nurses—Pat for my general clinic and Carolyn to run the IVF program. They were both compassionate, skilled nurses who always fought for the patients. They were both independent, not afraid to tell me what they thought. The three of us interacted along the gamut of emotions. We would sit and laugh during good times, cry together during bad times, and close the door and yell at each other if needed. I loved that quality in them. Having grown up with two feisty and independent women, my sister and mother, these two nurses were very comfortable for me. They kept me humble throughout many years. We built a cohesive team and began a journey of helping those in our area who were unable to conceive. We had a vision and a unified team. Our dream of building a program was coming true.

Even after 25 years, Pat and Carolyn remain very special to me. Carolyn, the IVF nurse, was in her 20s when she began working with me and knew nothing about infertility. But she brought a professionalism to the program as a high-level, well-trained ICU nurse. She saw me not as her boss but rather as her colleague, serving equally on the team. She knew her lane and stayed in it, and she knew my lane and kept me in it. It continues to be a fruitful partnership. Pat, my general nurse, was a pro in the field of infertility. She walked that fine line of taking orders from me while at the same time explaining "how things are typically done." She had a love for patients, and they instinctively knew it. Both Carolyn and Pat were able to successfully influence me, albeit in different ways. Carolyn's influence was through intellectualism and a forceful spirit, while Pat's was through a combination of loyalty, incredible experience, and a loving deference at times.

After six months of preparing to set up our protocols and the lab, we started two cycles in December 1990. Much to our delight, our first patient got pregnant and had a healthy delivery in 1991. We were off and running.

Quick success was wonderful but also brought a strong desire to make the next year even better. I didn't want anyone to think it was a fluke. And in my youth and inexperience, I became a little serious, believing that a failure would say something about me. Now I know with experience that failure is part of life. As a colleague once said, "If you've not had failure in medicine, you simply haven't done enough cases."

As I was starting to take myself a little too seriously, along came Michael and Denise. Michael was a resident at our institution, so he understood the great weight that had been placed on my shoulders. He was carefree and could make people feel comfortable around him. They knew I was young and inexperienced yet put their full faith for this important cycle into my hands. There was no one else who could help them since I was the only IVF provider in the entire region. It's easy to see how I could become a little too intense. The program's failure would be my failure, or so this young doctor thought.

I had not yet learned that it was not all about me. It's all too easy to assume that the entire world is on your shoulders and that you are responsible for everyone and everything. Life has a way of doing that—bills to pay, deadlines to meet, people to help, trials to face. Even though external pressures are abundant, many of us suffer more from internal pressure. We take life too seriously. Actually, we were designed for celebration and joy. Even in the midst of adversity and responsibility, joy should be our foundation for living life. An ability to see life as a blessing, to see life as an adventure, or to see life as a time of growth may be the difference between living life to the fullest and living life in fear, waiting for the next calamity. While there are times to be serious, there are also an abundance of times when it is important to find joy in the midst of trial.

Their cycle went well, and we came to the day for the actual embryo transfer. The embryo transfer is the emotional high-water mark of the cycle. It is the day patients are all waiting for, the day when embryos are placed into the uterus. For many women who don't have success, this is the day they often speak of fondly—the day when they were pregnant. We always try very hard to make this an extraordinary day.

Interestingly, in the early days of IVF, we didn't know if activity would lead to lower success rates. So after the embryo transfer, women would stay in bed for several hours with limited activity. I even remember using bedpans in those early days. But looking back, we now realize it was not all necessary.

Now back to the story. Since the embryo transfer is special, IVF providers work very hard to make the transfer of the embryos as smooth as possible. We don't want any bleeding, cramping, or mucous in the catheter. The catheter is very soft and specially designed to traverse the cervix and enter the uterine cavity without difficulty. Some cases take extra expertise and experience. We go through all those years of training to make sure the embryos slide in effortlessly and nestle into the uterine lining, implanting a couple of days later—no drama, no delays, no fuss. We always want the patient to feel like everything is going perfectly.

The transfer on Denise was perfect. Two embryos were easily placed. I backed away from the bed, looking very proud, and told her in no uncertain terms to lie as still as possible. My routine has always been to leave the couple alone for 20 to 30 minutes to allow them time to fully comprehend the moment, come a little closer together as a couple, and allow the embryos the best environment possible. They should look back on this moment with no regrets, positive pregnancy or not—a turning point in their lives, a movement from the pain of infertility to the next season of their life. Surely they felt and understood the seriousness of the day.

When I walked back roughly 30 minutes later, I was surprised and perplexed to find Denise writhing around on the bed, moaning as if in severe pain. What in the world was happening? I've never had a complication from an embryo transfer. The catheter was so soft that surely there was no way I could have damaged anything. And in the midst of this thought, I also began to worry about the process. If there is this much pain and movement, how can all our efforts of the past month lead to success? Though I hate to admit it, I was thinking, *How will this reflect on me?* Michael was trying to comfort Denise. I moved in quickly to her side, took her hand, and tried to comfort her, but I also tried to figure out what was going on.

At just the right moment, both Michael and Denise reached under the sheet between her legs to grab something. In a movement you only see in the delivery room, they proudly "delivered" two fully blown-up balloons, each with a face drawn on it. We all started laughing uncontrollably. Even I, all worried about the embryos (and myself), couldn't help but laugh. I immediately knew there was something special about this couple. After the mandatory time, we discharged the couple and planned for her pregnancy test roughly 11 days later. I tried to explain the emotional struggles of the next 11 days, the time when there may be a pregnancy but with no way to find out for sure—sort of a no man's land, guardedly optimistic, not knowing what to say to family or friends.

Not expecting to hear from them, I went about my business for the next several days. Six days after the transfer, too early to tell if the cycle had been successful, I received a call from Denise.

"We've been offered a newborn to adopt," she said, "and we have to decide today. What should we do?"

Wow! What are the odds of this timing? I knew they wanted a biological offspring; otherwise, why go through the IVF process? I also knew that most IVF cycles in these early days did not work. I began to inwardly struggle with what

I should say. I didn't want her to pass on the infant, have a negative pregnancy test, and languish in the pain of infertility. But I also didn't want to force her into an adoption with all its unique struggles. Sometimes there is no easy answer. And in those situations you can't control, it's always best to embrace whatever life gives you. Some would view this decision as a blessing while others might see it as a burden. I love partnering with couples who take the former approach, and I instinctively knew that Michael and Denise saw life as a blessing and were willing to fully enter into its ups and downs.

I said, "Statistically, you are likely not to be pregnant. If you are open to the concept of adoption, I'd take the baby."

They did. And five days later she found out that she was indeed pregnant. They welcomed the adopted daughter into their lives and delivered a healthy biological daughter nine months later—two girls, only a few months apart, raised as sisters. They were like twin girls from different mothers, bound in a very unique way to a new mother and father, both willing to embrace life fully.

Life can be hell with struggles coming from all directions. You may see your life as a burden, trying to hide as much as possible by keeping boundaries around your heart. I encourage you to see your life as a blessing, laughing at the most inopportune times and accepting a daughter into your life at a time when you are celebrating a long-awaited pregnancy. I'm so glad Denise and Michael took the latter view of life and taught a young, inexperienced doctor to lighten up and embrace life fully.

Dr. Deaton's Prescription: We read that a joyful heart does the body good, just like medicine. So, my prescription for you today is simple: Find ways to bring joy into your day. You don't have to look very hard, for joyful moments are all around you—your toddler singing to herself as she plays, a phone call from a friend, beautiful clouds overhead, a glass of wine shared with that most important person in your life.

As you recognize these joyful moments, take time to notice just how much better you feel. Refill this prescription as often as you like.

How will you follow this prescription?

UNDERSTANDING YOUR FIRST FERTILITY SPECIALIST VISIT

While each individual's journey is unique, the initial consultation with a fertility specialist often follows a similar structure, laying the groundwork for diagnosis and a personalized treatment plan. Expect this first appointment to last between 30 and 60 minutes and bringing your partner can be very beneficial. In recent times, virtual consultations via video have become common, offering greater convenience by allowing you to connect from work or home. This initial visit primarily involves discussion where you'll have the opportunity to ask questions and collaboratively develop a general plan. Come prepared with any questions you may have. A list can be helpful. This is your time to build comfort and trust with your doctor and fully understand the proposed plan, including the financial aspects. Ensure all your questions and concerns are addressed.

Your doctor will likely outline a series of tests, unless you've already completed them, and discuss some important issues to provide a comprehensive assessment and treatment plan. These tests typically include the following:

Semen Analysis: In heterosexual couples facing infertility, a male factor contributes to approximately 40% of cases. Therefore, a thorough evaluation of the male partner is crucial. While a comprehensive semen analysis involves numerous parameters, key indicators of normal function include the following:

- *Volume:* 1.5–5.0 milliliters (ml)
- *Sperm count:* At least 15 million sperm per milliliter (ml)
- *Motility:* At least 30% of sperm showing movement
- *Strict morphology:* At least 4% of sperm have a normal shape

Lifestyle modifications might improve a mild abnormality in sperm parameters. They include healthier habits such as more fruits and vegetables, exercise, and weight loss. Smoking, drug use, excessive alcohol use, and bodybuilding supplements have been shown to lower men's fertility. Your doctor may also recommend a referral to a urologist with special training in male factor infertility.

Evaluation of Ovulatory Cycles: Assessing whether you are ovulating regularly is a fundamental step. The hormone progesterone, crucial for the luteal phase of the menstrual cycle, is primarily produced by the corpus luteum, a temporary ovarian structure that forms after ovulation. Progesterone levels typically rise from a pre-ovulatory baseline (below 2.0 ng/ml) to a peak (above 10.0 ng/ml) approximately seven days after ovulation. Your fertility specialist will likely order a progesterone blood test, either on a specific day after suspected ovulation or timed using a urine ovulation predictor kit. Low progesterone levels can indicate an ovulatory disturbance, which is often treatable with fertility medications.

Ovarian Reserve Testing (Egg Number): Understanding the quantity of the remaining eggs is essential. The anti-Müllerian hormone (AMH) blood test serves as a key marker of ovarian reserve. Eggs develop early in fetal life, reaching their peak number (around seven million) at about five months of gestation. From that point onward, the number of eggs gradually declines until menopause. While a woman starts with millions of eggs, only about 400 will be ovulated throughout her reproductive years. Some individuals may naturally have a lower initial egg count, or their eggs may decline more rapidly, leading to variations in the age of menopause. Currently, there is no way to create new eggs, making ovarian reserve a critical factor in fertility treatment. A low AMH level can raise concerns about the potential for earlier menopause and a possible increased risk of miscarriage or embryo genetic abnormalities. AMH is produced by specific stages of developing follicles in the ovaries, making it a reliable indicator of ovarian reserve.

Uterine Cavity and Fallopian Tube Evaluation: Either a hysterosalpingogram (HSG) or a saline infusion sonohysterogram (SIS) will likely be recommended to assess the uterus and fallopian tubes. Fallopian tubes are vital for natural conception since they facilitate the meeting of sperm and egg. After ovulation, the egg enters the outer part of the tube (ampulla) and waits while sperm travel from the cervix through the uterus and into the tube to reach the egg for fertilization. The fertilized egg then travels back down the tube and implants in the uterus. Blocked fallopian tubes due to congenital issues, scar tissue, or pelvic infections can impede this process.

Hysterosalpingogram (HSG): This is an X-ray procedure often performed in the hospital where a dye is introduced into the uterus to visualize the uterine cavity for abnormalities such as polyps, fibroids, or scar tissue. The dye hopefully passes freely out of the ends of the fallopian tubes, indicating patency (openness).

Sonohysterogram (SIS): This procedure uses an ultrasound and a special fluid that enhances visualization and is done in the doctor's office. It is particularly effective for evaluating the uterine cavity and can also show if fluid passes through the fallopian tubes. While SIS is usually the preferred test due to its better evaluation of the uterus, HSG can provide a clearer view of tubal patency if this is of utmost importance to understand.

Discussion of Pelvic Pain, Intercourse Pain, or Abnormal Uterine Bleeding: While the aforementioned tests form the core of the initial workup, your doctor will also inquire about any pelvic pain, pain during intercourse, or abnormal uterine bleeding. Persistent pelvic pain can sometimes indicate underlying conditions such as pelvic endometriosis or scar tissue, which can be diagnosed and often treated with a minimally invasive outpatient surgical procedure called laparoscopy. Similarly, abnormal bleeding may suggest uterine fibroids or polyps, which can often be detected with SIS and treated with outpatient hysteroscopy. If surgery is deemed necessary, laparoscopy and hysteroscopy can often be performed simultaneously. Recovery is typically quick with most individuals returning to work within a week or even the next day for a hysteroscopy alone. If you are not experiencing these symptoms, surgery is usually not part of the initial evaluation.

Analysis of Insurance Coverage for Infertility: Fertility treatments can be a significant financial investment. So, understanding your insurance coverage is a crucial aspect of planning. While most insurance plans cover the initial diagnostic testing, coverage for treatments can vary widely, with some plans offering limited or no coverage for more advanced procedures. Your fertility specialist's office should have a financial counselor who can help you navigate your insurance benefits. If your plan lacks treatment coverage, there are potential avenues to explore. If your AMH levels are favorable, you might consider a period of financial planning to save for future treatments. Additionally, you may advocate for coverage with your company's human resources department since they often influence insurance decisions. Finally, researching companies in your area that offer comprehensive infertility coverage as part of their benefits package might be an option to consider if advanced treatment is necessary and financially challenging. It's important to remember that infertility is a medical condition and ideally should be covered by insurance, although that is not always the case.

While this overview provides a general understanding of what to expect, remember that individual experiences may vary. It's also important to know that approximately 10%–15% of couples may receive more than one diagnosis, which can present additional complexities. Even in these situations, one diagnosis often guides the treatment approach. Furthermore, in roughly 10% of cases, no diagnosis is found, leading to what is called unexplained infertility. Since you probably want to know what is causing your infertility, unexplained infertility can be a very frustrating situation. Don't be discouraged since there are good treatment options for unexplained infertility. If you are concerned about your out-of-pocket costs, remember that many individuals achieve pregnancy through simpler, office-based techniques that are not overly expensive.

Don't let fear of the unknown deter you from seeking help. For many, pursuing recommended treatments can ultimately lead to the fulfillment of their dream of parenthood. Take that courageous first step, seek out a fertility specialist, and address your fertility concerns. It could lead to the family you've always envisioned.

CHAPTER 6

DON'T STOP LIVING

I have always enjoyed gynecology because it allows me the privilege of locking arms with women to help them build families in the midst of adversity. Too often I see them despair over their infertility, often to the point of giving up on their dreams. Fortunately, early in my career, a 15-year-old girl taught me the value of living on purpose.

As a well-trained, board-certified fertility specialist, I had a large referral base for laparoscopic surgery, done through the belly button and an emerging field in the 1990s. Most well-trained laparoscopic surgeons at that time were infertility physicians. In my early days at Wake Forest, I was the person doing the aggressive surgery through the belly button, and many gynecologists sent me patients for this very reason.

I received a call from a colleague about a young girl with a pelvic infection. Katy, only 15, had been diagnosed with a bilateral tubal abscess. I took her to the operating room where she underwent a laparoscopy to determine the scope of the problem and repair her damaged tubes. While not surprised, I was distraught at the extent of her disease. Both tubes were filled with fluid, extremely dilated, and blocked. As a fertility physician, I quickly realized that her chance for a natural conception was extremely low. While not zero, it was close. Usually, with today's technology, we would remove the tubes and do IVF. But she was only 15 years old. And besides, IVF at that time was not very successful.

I took a deep breath, put on some music, often Ella Fitzgerald or Dire Straits, and went to work trying to repair her tubes. I cut the scar tissue, opened the tubes, and created new openings at the end of the tube near the ovaries. But a tube has a delicate end called the fimbria, the mechanism whereby an egg from the ovary is pulled into the tube in preparation for fertilization. Without fimbria, the chance of a natural conception is almost zero. And there were no fimbria present in either of Katy's tubes. But I persisted since the thought of telling a 15-year-old she cannot conceive naturally was too much for even me to bear.

After the surgery, I met with the family. They were full of optimism and thanked me for the work I performed. They didn't worry about Katy's fertility since their focus was on her health. That was the kind of love they had. Depriving Katy of a family was never in their thought process. Never did they despair, and I'm sure they took the same attitude around Katy.

As a gynecologist, I'm not typically working with parents, but this was refreshing in one way because they were a supportive family. Katy's ability to bear children did not change their love for her or their ability to parent her. But it was challenging since they were now facing the fact that Katy's life would be forever changed. Would she despair and turn toward an unfulfilled life? Would she ever rebound from this major life event? Would she find a partner who would love her purely for herself? Would infertility destroy her relationships? I knew all these potential pitfalls, but Katy's parents seemed to not focus on these outcomes. They simply loved her.

I lost touch with Katy and her family for about 15 years. I never really knew how they approached her infertility, but I bet they loved her unconditionally and kept encouraging her. I bet they assured her of her worth, even though she might not be able to have a child. I bet they spoke of her purpose and told her to seize life for all it has to offer. I can say that now, and here's why.

I was having a typical day seeing new patients when my nurse brought me a chart on a 30-year-old woman named Katy. I walked in the room to find a delightful young woman with a smile spread across her face. She spoke of the surgery 15 years earlier and went on to explain that both of her tubes had been removed in a later operation. She understood that her only chance of a successful pregnancy was through IVF. She approached the conversation with confidence and a demeanor that exuded self-worth.

She was spunky, the kind of attitude that had grown from a base of self-confidence. I learned that she was a successful lawyer, had a great marriage to Kevin, and was part of a church that gathered around and supported infertility couples. Becoming a lawyer seemed perfect for her, and I knew I would not like to face her in court unless she were on my side.

Her church also seemed special. They gathered around and supported infertile couples in their congregation. No condemnation. No judgment. No pointing fingers at perceived sins. Just love and support. This is rare but is a hallmark of a good church. Many in churches look for causes of an illness, quick to point a finger and encourage repentance, but not this church. They loved instead.

Katy was not only living life, but she was also embracing it fully, not willing to let anything deter her from her destiny. I found myself encouraged simply being in her presence. She was a victor, regardless of her circumstances.

We embarked on her IVF journey. Unfortunately, a blood test revealed her egg quality was diminished, which meant that the success rate of IVF was markedly lowered. We also learned that her insurance company was not going to pay for the cycle. But even in the face of these two significant disappointments, she was not deterred. She moved forward with optimism.

Her husband, Kevin, was perfect for her. He was always happy and managed to cheer us up during some of the difficult conversations. He also had faith, never doubting their eventual outcome. They would banter back and forth in a way that seemed perfect. I could never tell which one was really in charge—perhaps neither. But it was fun and a delight to watch.

Her IVF cycle had the typical ups and downs—the emotional roller coaster of IVF. After multiple daily shots, several mature eggs developed, and she underwent an uneventful egg retrieval. But we only got six eggs. Again, she handled the disappointment well. After fertilization, we were delighted to have five good embryos, and one was placed in her uterus five days after the egg retrieval. One of the remaining embryos did not develop to the freezing stage, and three were frozen for later use. Now we were all expectant of a good outcome. Eight days later, her pregnancy test came back positive.

It's hard to imagine the emotions she must have felt. Since the age of 15, she had faced the fact that getting pregnant would not be easy. One of the most important moments of a person's life—the birth of a child—should not be accompanied by heartache. But isn't it true that dreams are often realized after long journeys through peaks and valleys? She spent 15 years wondering about her fertility, and now she was pregnant. Some would say that 15 years as a young woman, wondering every day if she would be able to become a mother, must have seemed painfully slow. For Katy, I wonder if the years flew by because she chose to keep living.

I always repeat the pregnancy test one week later to make sure the level is rising normally. When the nurse told me the level had dropped, my heart sank. Katy was going to have a miscarriage. While I understood that her miscarriage was unrelated to her pelvic infection as a young girl, I worried that she would try to link the two. But she didn't. While I'm sure there were some private moments of grief, her public persona was upbeat.

She took a break for a while. Both she and her husband took new jobs. I'm sure they felt the need to do something to regain control of this most important part of their young marriage. I knew that control is ultimately an illusion, but I'm sure it helped them to reboot their lives.

Not much later, she came back for another try, and we placed two thawed embryos into her uterus. When the pregnancy test came back positive, we were all happy but a bit more hesitant than the first time. Guarded optimism is much more common after a prior miscarriage. Once again, much to our sorrow, she miscarried. While I became more concerned about this young couple's emotional state, Katy and Kevin remained upbeat.

After another break, she came back for one final try with her only remaining frozen embryo. She was honest—this would be her very last try. As a more seasoned infertility doctor, I was better able to handle this than I would have earlier in my practice. But I was still a young man. The pressure of the "last try" was intense. We prepared her uterus and synchronized it to the age of the embryo. The embryo was thawed and transferred into her uterus. Eight days later, once again we found a positive pregnancy test. The emotions were guarded, and we all began the long waiting game.

One week later, the levels looked great. We remained guarded but hopeful. How must Katy be feeling? I wish I could understand better how women feel during this time of waiting. Guarded optimism? Hopeful pessimism? Happily nervous? I bet all women are a little different.

But I do know how it feels to be denied the one thing a heart desires. When that happened in my life, it made me feel small. It made me feel unqualified. It made me feel like there was nothing special in me. It made me feel like I had no purpose on this earth. It made me feel unloved in a grand sort of way. Did Katy also have these feelings? If she did, they were kept in the recesses of her heart.

All these emotions are very normal, but I've seen too many women get stuck in despair and lose hope. If I could be given a special superpower, it might be to share this with each one of them: You are unique, you are blessed, you are loved, you have a purpose on this earth. I have always believed that to be the truth, no matter the circumstances of a seemingly hopeless existence.

Katy showed up two weeks later for her ultrasound, and there on that tiny black and white screen for all to see was a fetus and a healthy heartbeat. Katy was going to be a mother! Kevin was going to be a father! The enormity of the past 15 years began to settle in. I had prepared Katy for a possible adoption or child-free living, so I knew she would be okay regardless of the outcome. That is always part of my job—to shepherd a couple's emotions through this tumultuous season as they journey toward a family.

Of course, Katy wanted a child, but her life was not defined by this single blessing. She knew who she was and what she was worth. While challenging, she would have handled the loss of her dream for a pregnancy. This one dream did not define her. There were many others. I will always credit her family and her husband for believing in her. It's impossible to develop this type of self-worth in isolation.

We are all here for a purpose, but it's very easy to get derailed and off track in life. When you're hit with something difficult, does it redefine your life? Or is it merely a boulder in the road along the journey, something you just need to go around, something that causes a minor detour? Don't let a major disappointment or trial get you off track. You have a purpose. Stay on the journey.

The enormity of treating her as a 15-year-old and then coming full circle to help her have a child began to settle into a physician's heart. I have learned to face and handle great adversity, and I've also learned to celebrate on the pinnacle of success. And this felt like Mount Everest.

Some dreams come true within moments of dreaming. Others can take 15 years or longer, like the birth of this precious boy. Try to find the balance, keep dreaming, and keep living your life, even during the seasons of suffering. Try to grow, like Katy, during the waiting.

Even though this one little girl's hopes and dreams took many years to come true, holding and raising Samuel made all the waiting worth it. So many years is a long time to wait, but it's a great celebration when waiting becomes life.

Dr. Deaton's Prescription: Here is your prescription. It is to be taken daily, even hourly, without fail. I am writing this prescription to help keep you living in times of despair, to help you keep dreaming when it seems there is only darkness, to help you know there is so much more to who you are than you can even imagine.

I want you to embrace hope. It may be all that gets you out of bed and keeps you going. Never let go. No matter your disappointments, no matter your fears or failures, never let go. You are special. You are blessed. You are loved. And you do have a great purpose in this life.

If you're having a tough time, think of someone who has brought hope into your life. Call or write to them. Thank them and see if they can do it again.

How will you follow this prescription?

NAVIGATING THE INITIAL INFERTILITY TREATMENT PLANS

Once your infertility evaluation is complete, you and your partner will likely receive a specific diagnosis or fall into a category that guides the next steps. Most couples will have a single diagnosis. While the science and emotional aspects of infertility can feel overwhelming, the initial approach generally falls into one of a few key treatment plans. Here's an overview of common infertility diagnoses and their typical first-line treatments.

Female Ovulation Disorders: Many women experience infrequent or absent ovulation. If you ovulate less than once a month or not at all, your physician will likely recommend a hormonal evaluation. That may involve testing a few key hormones—prolactin, thyroid-stimulating hormone (TSH)—and a pregnancy test or a more comprehensive panel that assesses the function of the pituitary and adrenal glands. Depending on your specific situation, your doctor may also check pituitary hormones—follicle-stimulating hormone (FSH) and luteinizing hormone (LH)—and male hormones (in cases of abnormal hair growth). They may screen for insulin resistance or diabetes. Once the underlying cause of the ovulation disorder is identified, appropriate medication can often be prescribed. If no other fertility factors are present, these medications alone can lead to high success rates. Some common reasons for ovulation disorders and their initial management include the following:

- *High Prolactin:* An elevated prolactin level will typically be retested while fasting. If it remains high, a brain MRI may be ordered to check for a small, prolactin-producing tumor. Once the cause is identified, prolactin levels can usually be effectively managed with medications called dopamine agonists, often leading to resumption of menses and fertility.

- *Abnormal TSH:* A mildly elevated TSH, especially in the presence of thyroid antibodies, might prompt your doctor to initiate thyroid medication. Significantly low or high TSH levels will likely warrant a referral to a Medical Endocrinologist for specialized management.

- *High FSH:* If your FSH level is consistently elevated above 40 mIU/ml on two separate tests approximately two weeks apart, it strongly suggests menopause. For women under 35, this finding will trigger a more extensive evaluation to determine the cause of premature menopause. If menopause is the diagnosis, your doctor will discuss the option of using donor eggs since your own egg supply is depleted.

- *Low FSH and LH:* Some women experience hypothalamic amenorrhea, a condition often linked to intense exercise, significant stress, and low body fat (sometimes associated with eating disorders). A single condition in excess (e.g., anorexia) or a combination of two or three of these factors can contribute to this condition. While oral medications might be an option, injectable FSH (gonadotropins) are often the most effective treatment. Due to the increased risk of multiple births in younger women with this condition, some may choose to proceed directly to IVF where the multiple birth risk can be managed. Gonadotropin therapy is costly and also carries risks, so it should only be administered under the close supervision of a fertility specialist.

- *High Male Hormones (Androgens):* Elevated androgen levels may indicate polycystic ovarian syndrome (PCOS) or an adrenal disorder, prompting further evaluation.
- *PCOS:* This is a very common hormonal disorder characterized by infrequent ovulation and infertility. In young women, PCOS is the diagnosis found in roughly 75% of patients who don't ovulate regularly. Common features of PCOS include obesity, abnormal hair growth or high serum androgens, the presence of multiple small follicles (at least 15 in each ovary), mildly elevated LH levels, high AMH, and insulin resistance. Roughly a third of PCOS patients do not suffer from obesity, so don't be fooled into thinking you need to be obese to have PCOS. Initial treatment for PCOS often involves oral fertility medications such as the following:
  - » *Letrozole:* This aromatase inhibitor lowers estrogen levels, which in turn stimulates the pituitary to release FSH, encouraging follicle growth and egg maturation. The risk of twins with letrozole is around 8%, and triplets are rare (under 1%). Most fertility specialists start with a dose of 5 mg per day on cycle days 3–7 and often perform an ultrasound around day 11 to monitor follicle development. If a dominant follicle is present with appropriate hormone levels, an injection of hCG (the "trigger shot") is often administered to mimic the LH surge,

triggering ovulation, increasing progesterone, and promoting final egg maturation. Following the trigger shot, couples are typically advised to have intercourse one to two times during the fertile window.

» *Clomiphene Citrate:* This older fertility drug works by blocking the effects of estrogen, also leading to an increase in FSH release. It is administered and monitored similarly to letrozole and has a comparable multiple birth rate.

Male Factor Infertility: Approximately 30%–40% of infertility cases involve abnormal sperm parameters. If a significant male factor is suspected, your fertility doctor will likely recommend that the male partner consult with a urologist who specializes in male infertility. This is important in order to rule out any treatable medical conditions or anatomical issues contributing to low sperm counts. Depending on the severity of the male factor, treatment options often include the following:

• *Intrauterine Insemination (IUI):* This procedure often involves the female partner taking a mild oral fertility medication like letrozole, followed by an hCG trigger shot to induce ovulation. Approximately 36–40 hours after the trigger, a sperm sample (either brought by the partner or collected in the office) is washed, and at least 5 million motile sperm are resuspended in a sperm-friendly media and gently inserted into the upper part of the uterus with a thin catheter, thus bypassing the cervix. For most women, this is a relatively simple and painless procedure. The pregnancy rate with IUI is around 30% over three attempts when there is only a mild male factor diagnosis.

- *In Vitro Fertilization (IVF):* Since IUI requires a certain number of motile sperm, cases of severe male factor need to consider IVF. This more advanced treatment option will be discussed in detail in a later chapter.

Tubal Disease: Blocked fallopian tubes, often resulting from previous pelvic infections such as chlamydia, are typically diagnosed during an HSG or SIS. For most women with tubal disease, IVF is the most effective treatment option. Other approaches have significantly lower success rates and can lead to ectopic pregnancies. If the female partner has a good ovarian reserve (AMH level), IVF outcomes are generally very favorable. However, if IVF is not a viable option due to cost or other reasons, consider these alternative approaches:

- *Proximal Tubal Blockage:* If the blockage is near the uterus, it may be possible to use a wire guided through the uterus to try to open the tubes. Discuss the availability of this procedure with your doctor.
- *Distal Tubal Blockage:* If the blockage is at the end of the fallopian tube near the ovary, surgery might be an option. However, success rates are typically low, and the risk of ectopic pregnancy is increased after such a surgery. Most women opt for IVF, but if it's not an option, discuss the potential benefits and risks of surgery with your doctor.

- *Tubal Ligation:* If you've had a tubal ligation, IVF is often the most effective path to pregnancy. In some cases where only a small portion of the tubes have been damaged, surgical reversal, called a tubal anastomosis, might be possible. However, success rates are generally lower than with IVF, and the risk of ectopic pregnancy is much higher. Discuss this option with your fertility specialist if you wish to avoid IVF.

Diminished Ovarian Reserve (Low AMH): A low AMH level doesn't necessarily equate to infertility, but it may indicate a shorter window of time to conceive. If you are not inclined to continue trying naturally, you might choose to pursue IVF to expedite the process and potentially bank embryos for future pregnancies. Given the current inability to create new eggs, embryo banking can be a valuable strategy for those with a low AMH who desire more than one child since frozen embryos do not age and the uterus remains capable of carrying a pregnancy for many years. It's crucial to have your AMH level interpreted by your fertility specialist as the report might say "normal," but ranges are highly age-dependent.

Pelvic Disease (Endometriosis or Scar Tissue): If the pelvic anatomy is distorted by conditions such as endometriosis or scar tissue, it can impede the egg's ability to enter the fallopian tube and be fertilized. Endometriosis, a condition where the uterine lining that sheds every month also implants outside the uterus, can be silent, and is often found in infertile women when the rest of the workup is normal. Common symptoms include worsening menstrual cramps as you age, pain during intercourse, bowel issues around menstruation, and premenstrual spotting. If these symptoms significantly impact your daily life, endometriosis can be diagnosed and often treated with outpatient laparoscopic surgery. Endometriosis has a familial tendency, so it may be helpful to inquire about its presence in your mother or sisters. While surgical treatment of endometriosis may not guarantee pregnancy, it can often alleviate associated symptoms. Laparoscopy is not a routine part of the infertility workup but is often recommended when significant symptoms are present.

Inadequate Exposure to Sperm: While sounding odd, this is a genuine reason why some individuals and couples seek fertility care. Examples include the following:

- Same-sex couples desiring pregnancy
- Erectile dysfunction
- Couples frequently apart during the woman's fertile window (due to travel or living arrangements)
- Single women desiring pregnancy

For these situations, IUI as described earlier is often the first-line treatment. While IUI has modest success rates in cases of male factor infertility, it can be highly effective when the primary issue is sperm not reaching the egg at the right time, such as in cases described above. Most pregnancies with IUI in these circumstances occur within the first three to four attempts. If IUI is unsuccessful, more aggressive treatments may be considered. Single women and same-sex couples will need to utilize sperm donation services, often through national sperm banks. Your doctor can recommend reputable sperm banks where you can purchase donor sperm.

Unexplained Infertility: Approximately 10%–15% of couples will receive a diagnosis of unexplained infertility. That doesn't mean there isn't a reason, but rather current medical knowledge hasn't identified it. This diagnosis can be frustrating for couples who understandably want to know the cause of their difficulties. Fortunately, treatments for unexplained infertility can be quite effective. The initial approach often involves letrozole combined with IUI, with a pregnancy rate of around 30% over three cycles. Couples who don't conceive with IUI, have a low AMH, or have good insurance coverage often move to IVF.

One more comment about unexplained infertility. Studies show that at least 60% of these women have minimal or mild endometriosis, which is often asymptomatic. Most fertility doctors do not put these women through surgery but recommend IUI followed by IVF. However, women who can't proceed to IVF often consider a diagnostic laparoscopy. If endometriosis is found and treated at surgery, roughly 30% of these women will conceive naturally in the six months following surgery if there is no other infertility factor. If surgery is completed and no pregnancy occurs in the six months after surgery, then you should consider moving to IVF.

A Final Note on Insurance: Every fertility specialist's office should have an insurance and financial specialist. It is crucial to work closely with this individual to understand your insurance coverage and the costs associated with your recommended treatment plan. Your financial situation is a significant factor in making informed decisions about your care. For example, if you have a diagnosis of low AMH, male factor infertility, or pelvic disease *and* have good insurance coverage, proceeding directly to IVF might be a more efficient option. While other treatments might be less costly initially, they are also less effective and could potentially delay your journey to parenthood. The goal is not only to help you achieve pregnancy but also to do so within your desired time frame. Don't hesitate to advocate for a more aggressive treatment approach if it aligns with your family-building goals and financial resources.

CHAPTER 7

IT NEVER HURTS TO ASK

I t has been a joy to watch my field of study and practice grow over the past 30 years. Think about it. Before 1978, there were no IVF babies. By 2024, 2.5% of all children born in the United States were conceived through IVF. Inseminations were first done in the 1960s. Before that, women were confined to achieving pregnancy only through the act of intercourse. They needed someone else. Now, women are free to pursue nontraditional forms of pregnancy. No longer are they dependent on a man to achieve a pregnancy. But this freedom was not easy.

I first met Maria in the late 1990s. My program was established, and we were experiencing great success. The institution was happy. My boss was delighted. All was well. On a typical clinic day, decisions were easy, and patients were content. I was content too. But I was also bothered that my superiors would not allow the insemination of single women. How could we deny them this service? I had to admit to a bit of conflict in my soul because I know the importance of a good dad. So I let this important issue lie dormant. I was nervous to rock the boat.

Then one day Maria came to see me. She was at peace, highly successful, delightful, and involved in a very long-term, same-sex relationship. A confident leader at her institution, she was accustomed to winning—and losing—battles. She knew how to embrace conflict if needed. Furthermore, at this time (prior to the Supreme Court ruling) states did not recognize same-sex relationships as married. Therefore, Maria was single in the eyes of the state.

During our 45-minute new patient appointment, I came to really like her. She was engaging, thoughtful, and drew me into her life. While content and satisfied, she and her partner wanted to welcome a child into their lives, not out of emptiness but out of fullness. There was no question in my mind that the child would be loved and nurtured. In fact, they had already discussed who would be the father figure to the child.

They were not looking to force social change or take this issue to the courts. They were not activists in the typical sense of the word. But their calm and professional demeanor coupled with their intelligence and sense of right and wrong led to activity on my part. I couldn't tell her that we don't inseminate single women. I took another approach and said, "This institution needs to address this issue. Do you mind if I take your case up to higher authorities?" To no surprise, she was okay with this approach. Conflict was her friend. They would be fine if we said no, so why not? They could always go to another facility in another part of the state.

I made an appointment to meet with our institutional chief of staff. He had been in charge for many, many years and was highly respected by all. In his 60s, he had white hair and a big gut. He smoked nonstop and spoke with a gruffness that made you listen. He was a classic old-school surgeon, and no one challenged him. As a young faculty member, I was scared of him. In fact, I tried to never cross his path. He had the authority and power to chew me up and spit me out.

I entered his office, and in his gruff and to-the-point style, he said, "Jeff, what can I do for you?" I tripped over my words, quickly showing my conflict about bringing a child into this world without a dad. I wonder if he even really knew what I was asking of him. He was very powerful in the church but had never really thought about this issue. He was taken a bit off guard.

Finally, after a few confusing minutes and with a lump in my throat, I said, "Can I see the policy that refuses the insemination of single women?" He looked at me, his hair a mess and a cigarette in one hand, and said, "We don't have a policy on that. We would rather not have anything in writing about that issue." I'm sure I had a stunned look on my face. Really? We had another short discussion about changing times and the ethics of denying women this care. We both agreed that it was not an easy decision, and I could be criticized for taking this path. He knew me reasonably well, quickly grasped the conflict, and decided to take the courageous path. He also knew he might be called to defend me with the institution's older established leadership. He finally said, "Do what you think is right."

I walked out of his office, slept on it, and changed the policy the next day. And immediately I felt a huge weight come off my shoulders. While the issue may be complex and I can respect opinions on both sides, in my heart I was feeling judgmental. That is why I so quickly changed the policy. People still ask me how I can justify inseminating single women when I so greatly value the presence of a father. There are two main reasons.

First, I realize I have been given a special place in society to walk with people through this most intimate of moments. Society has entrusted me with this position. My service is to all society, not just those with similar backgrounds. If I deny someone care while helping others, I am no longer serving society. I also don't want to get even close to being judgmental. Second, who am I to say who will be a good parent? If I start down this road, I might begin to judge almost everyone. Parenting is exquisitely complex. I've seen the best of parents struggle, and I've seen marginal parents raise exceptional children. So the weight came off my shoulders in an instant, thanks to Maria.

Maria and her partner, Rose, were happy with the decision, not because they wanted to be trailblazers but because they could now get on with their life. They picked an anonymous donor through one of the sperm banks and had the specimens shipped to my clinic to be placed in our sperm bank. Maria was extremely athletic and very thin, a combination that often leads to a lack of ovulation. In this group of people, the simpler oral fertility drugs often do not work. I had to move to the more complex and risky fertility injections. They are much more costly, cause a high rate of multiple births, and can lead to a dangerous condition called ovarian hyperstimulation syndrome.

In this syndrome, women's blood vessels become leaky, and they collect fluid in their abdominal cavity and occasionally in their chest cavity. They can develop severe dehydration and an imbalance in their electrolytes, which can be very dangerous and require hospitalization. Furthermore, the condition is exacerbated by pregnancy. It is caused by the development of too many eggs, so we often try very hard to limit the medicine and only get two to three eggs. In some women, this is not easy. Ovaries can be very sensitive to the medicine, leading to multiple eggs, multiple births, and hyperstimulation.

Maria's cycle went very well, but there were a few too many eggs, which led to a nervous doctor. But we decided to go ahead, and the insemination was easy. A few days after the insemination, she developed classic symptoms of hyperstimulation—enlarged ovaries, pelvic pain, and fluid in her pelvis. I knew that hyperstimulation tended to slowly get worse when there was an early pregnancy, but it was too early to do a pregnancy test.

If fluid accumulates in the pelvis, it can lead to severe discomfort and trouble breathing. This was beginning to happen to Maria. Fortunately, her blood electrolytes were stable, so I withdrew a lot of the fluid using a needle. In my experience, this often gives relief for three or so days. Maria was in excellent shape, but she was tiny and had no room to spare. The next day, she called me again and needed another needle drainage of new fluid. I knew this could potentially last a couple of weeks, so I prepared her for more drainage procedures.

Maria was used to getting her way and said, "We have a ski trip planned to Colorado. You need to do something so I can go." I knew these cases needed to stay around to get labs and fluid drainage every few days because hyperstimulation can be very dangerous. Maria persisted. Much to my shock, I offered a solution that I had never offered before and have not offered since. I said, "I guess I could put a drain in and let you drain the fluid off every day or two. But no skiing, and you can't get in the water."

Even though the words came out of my mouth, I began to question my thought process. What was I saying? The risk of infection is significant, and to my knowledge, no one had ever done this before. Maria proved she wanted to be the first, so why not? I put the drain in, sutured it to her skin, and taught her how to withdraw fluid and take care of it to prevent infection. She went off on her trip, had a great time, and took good care of the drain. On her return, her hyperstimulation was waning, and I removed the drain.

As expected, her pregnancy test was positive. She had a wonderful pregnancy and delivered a beautiful boy roughly eight months later. They were happy. I was delighted to help them achieve this goal and at the same time was content to have partnered with Maria to change a policy that was not right for the times.

I was glad to partner with Maria by taking a risk, challenging conventional thinking, and embarking on new experiences. We should be willing to think outside the box to help those in need. But my first-time experience with Maria did not end with the birth of her son. Shortly before his birth, she found herself coaching her team in a critical match. I decided to watch the game that was occurring in her home stadium. Much to everyone's delight, except of course the opposing team players, Maria's team won. They were champions.

Everyone was leaving the stadium, and the players were also emptying out. I was sitting there enjoying the sunshine of a beautiful fall day. From the field, I heard someone yell, "Dr. Deaton! Is that you?" I looked down, and there stood Rose with a huge smile on her face. She then yelled, "Come on down and join the celebration!" I walked down the steps and sort of jumped onto the field. Rose then escorted me across the field and to the third floor of the sports complex. We made our way down the hall into a room of roughly 12 female college athletes, a couple of trainers, and Maria. The room was electric. Maria hugged me and introduced me to several of the players. Of course, they were focused on being champions.

For the next hour or so, I celebrated with her championship team. I pondered the intersection of our lives. I realized how blessed I was to share in the most intimate moment of their lives. I was celebrating a championship only because our lives crossed in a most unique and unexpected way. These experiences of bonding with someone in their time of need and helping them fulfill a dream have led to incredibly unique relationships that have enlarged me and brought a fullness into my life.

And it all happened simply because Maria and Rose were willing to ask a hard question. If you are facing a tough decision and need an answer to a difficult question, it never hurts to ask. I learned it is always best to try to say yes. You may find yourself popping champagne in the midst of a championship celebration.

Dr. Deaton's Prescription: Risk-taking is necessary in life if we are ever to grow and mature. It is a risk to give your heart to someone in love. It is a risk to bring a child into the world. It is a risk to let your children—when they reach a certain age—go off and live their lives independently. And yet often the greater the risk, the greater the reward.

Think about a decision or action you have been putting off because of the risk. Determine today to set your fears aside, follow your heart, and walk boldly.

How will you follow this prescription?

FAMILY BUILDING WHEN YOU IDENTIFY AS LGBTQ+

We navigate a world with both encouraging progress and disheartening setbacks. The increasing societal acceptance of same-sex marriage was a significant step forward. However, recent challenges in healthcare for transgender individuals remind us that the journey toward full equality and affirmation continues. While a deep dive into these broader issues isn't the focus here, it's crucial to acknowledge the evolving landscape. As the percentage of people in our country who identify as LGBTQ+ (now over 10%) increases, my hope is that we will see continued and consistent progress in inclusive healthcare, including fertility care.

If you identify as LGBTQ+ and are on the path to building your family through fertility treatments, please know this: The vast majority of fertility specialists have been welcoming and treating LGBTQ+ individuals and couples for many years and are very comfortable providing care in this area. Furthermore, their offices are generally committed to being LGBTQ+ friendly spaces. My sincere hope is that you find a safe and affirming environment for your fertility journey.

The history of LGBTQ+ individuals seeking fertility care dates back to the widespread use of insemination in the 1970s and 1980s when same-sex female couples began seeking out specialists to start their families. This history is a key reason why most fertility providers are experienced and at ease working with LGBTQ+ patients. Initially, many donor sperm inseminations were done with "fresh" samples. However, due to concerns about HIV and other STIs, government regulations were implemented. Currently, all donor sperm is frozen and quarantined, allowing time for the donor to be retested for STIs. Only if the donor remains negative is the sperm released for use in insemination. Current practices involve IUI with thoroughly washed sperm where at least eight million motile sperm are isolated and frozen for purchase and later use. The development of sperm-freezing techniques and governmental oversight over the past 25 years has led to the growth of numerous sperm banks catering to these needs.

While a fertility specialist will address many important aspects of your care, these three foundational questions apply to everyone but are particularly relevant for LGBTQ+ individuals and couples:

- Who will provide the egg?
- Who will provide the sperm?
- Who will provide the uterus?

For Same-Sex Female Couples: Typically, there are ample eggs and two potential uteri, but access to sperm requires assistance through a sperm donor. The crucial decision is who will provide the egg and who will carry the pregnancy. If one partner provides both the egg and carries the pregnancy (and is fertile), simple IUIs using donor sperm offer very high success rates. The IUI process is straightforward, involving an ultrasound to monitor egg development, a trigger shot to induce ovulation, and a final, usually painless insemination procedure where a small catheter delivers 8–10 million washed sperm directly into the upper part of the uterus. There are typically no activity restrictions following an IUI. If three to four IUIs are unsuccessful, further diagnostic tests or more advanced treatment protocols can be considered.

The next key decision is selecting a sperm source. Most same-sex female couples purchase donor sperm from established sperm banks. Your provider can offer guidance on the banks they work with and the process of donor matching. Choosing a donor can be a quick process or may take more time, depending on the importance of specific criteria for you. Using a known sperm donor is also an option. However, your fertility clinic will need to adhere to all government regulations, including sperm quarantine and STI testing, which can take time. If using a known donor is important, plan accordingly and allow ample time for this process. Many couples appreciate the idea of a known donor as it can feel important to have a familiar male figure in their child's life. This process also involves legal contracts between the couple and the donor, so discuss potential attorneys who can assist your clinic with this.

Finally, reciprocal IVF is an important option for same-sex female couples. If one partner provides both the egg and the uterus, the other partner may feel less connected to the pregnancy. Reciprocal IVF allows one partner to provide the egg, which is then fertilized with donor sperm, and the other partner carries the pregnancy. For a second child, the partners can switch roles. That allows both partners to feel a biological connection to the pregnancy, with one contributing the genetic material and the other nurturing the pregnancy. Discuss reciprocal IVF with your provider if this interests you. While technically manageable for the clinic, it's important to note that it involves two separate IVF cycles and is therefore more expensive.

For Same-Sex Male Couples: Typically, there is readily available sperm, but access to eggs and a uterus requires assistance. Your role in the initial stages is often simpler and focuses on selecting an appropriate egg donor. Similar to sperm donation, egg donors are found through egg banks. Young women are recruited to donate their eggs, and these egg banks provide catalogs with donor profiles for you to review. You can often search based on criteria that are important to you and typically purchase a cohort of six to eight eggs at a time. This number usually results in two to three viable embryos. The primary consideration here is cost as donor eggs can be expensive. Using a known egg donor is also possible but is a more complex and costly undertaking. If you have someone, typically under the age of 30, you'd like to consider as an egg donor, discuss it with your provider.

Once you've chosen an egg donor, the next step is finding a uterus to carry the pregnancy—a gestational carrier. That can be legally and emotionally complex as it involves asking another woman to carry a pregnancy for nine months, deliver the baby, and then relinquish parenthood. If you don't have someone in mind, there are agencies that specialize in matching intended parents with gestational carriers, but that can be very expensive. If you know someone who might be willing to serve as a gestational carrier, discuss it with your provider so the gestational carrier can undergo the necessary screening, including psychological counseling and legal contracts. While this process may seem daunting, most fertility clinics have personnel, often called third-party reproduction coordinators, who can guide you through each step.

For Transgender Men: Many transgender men desire children and want genetic continuity with their offspring. As someone born with ovaries and a uterus, it's important to reach out to a fertility center before undergoing pelvic surgery to remove these organs. Current technology makes it relatively easy to undergo ovarian stimulation followed by egg retrieval and egg freezing. That allows you to preserve your eggs for future use and ensures a genetic link to your child.

Many transgender men after egg freezing wish to proceed with pelvic surgery and do not desire to carry a pregnancy themselves. The decision of where to obtain sperm and a uterus depends on their partner. If the transgender man has a male partner, sperm is readily available, and they will need to find a gestational carrier. If the transgender man has a female partner, a uterus is likely available, and they can utilize donor sperm to fertilize their frozen eggs.

For Transgender Women: Preserving sperm for future use is a straightforward and relatively inexpensive process for transgender women prior to undergoing orchiectomy (removal of the testicles). If you are considering this and desire genetic continuity with your future children, please speak with a fertility clinic as soon as possible.

While this overview cannot cover every specific situation, please know that IVF centers are equipped to help you navigate all these pathways. As with heterosexual couples, you have the fundamental right to procreate and build your family. Do not hesitate to advocate for these rights. Any reputable IVF center in the United States should be comfortable assisting with donor sperm, donor eggs, gestational carriers, and all the associated psychological and legal considerations. While it may feel overwhelming at times, remember that IVF centers are experts in this area and have dedicated personnel to help you achieve your dream of parenthood. I wish you the very best on your journey.

CHAPTER 8

THE GIFT OF ENCOURAGEMENT

I will never forget my third-year medical school clerkship in obstetrics and gynecology at Vanderbilt. My mentor was Dr. Anne Colston Wentz, one of the most prominent reproductive endocrinologists in the country. She built a top-notch team in an attempt to successfully conceive the first IVF baby in the United States. The first IVF baby in the world was born in England in 1978 under the direction of Drs. Steptoe and Edwards, which later led to a Nobel Prize. Of course, there were many others on this historic team, including Jean Purdy who served tirelessly for many years as their research and clinical nurse.

No one had yet been successful in the United States. Dr. Wentz was poised to make history, and I was a third-year medical student wanting to be part of that history. I was already drawn to Ob/Gyn, and I also considered pursuing infertility because of Dr. Wentz's influence on my life. I spent a summer doing research with her, so I was pulling for her and the team at Vanderbilt.

As a student, I was only on the periphery of the intensity. Dr. Wentz loved students and loved teaching, and she was caught in this endeavor for the first IVF baby in the United States. She was truly a pioneer, only one of a few women in academic leadership positions in the country. She was a wonderful role model for a young medical student.

In the 1970s, and 1980s, women were coming into spheres of influence and leadership in ways never before seen. I had grown up around strong women, not the least of which were my mother and older sister. As a Southern boy coming of age at that time, I was able to observe all kinds of women. I watched women who felt that the highest calling for a woman was to be a good homemaker, spouse, and mother. That remains a high calling. I watched other women who perhaps wanted to enter the workforce but decided against it due to the difficulties of navigating a male-dominated environment.

As the 1980s progressed, I was able to observe up close those women who entered the workforce who wanted to make professional environments a better place for women. Being in academic medicine, I was also able to observe a few women who dreamed of running a large academic medical school department, equal in authority to the male leaders of the day. Anne Colston Wentz was one of those women.

She was not an activist or demonstrator; instead, she led by example. One of few women professors at Vanderbilt, she stood out. While 5' 5" with short, cropped hair, she seemed much taller to this young student and was always the dominant presence in the room due to her keen intellect and her flamboyant and emotional delivery style. While never loud, you always knew where she stood on an issue. She was determined to be seen as decisive. She always wore a dress.

Having a solid background in feminism through my mom and my sister, I was now able to watch the next level up close. Dr. Wentz walked the corridors of power during a time when many men in leadership did not know what to do with a female in authority. It was fun to watch. As a woman who saw herself as a leader, she was able to constantly keep powerful men on guard. They didn't know how to handle this new phenomenon. Her intellect was delightful to observe but could be brutal at times. During rounds when the residents would present patients, Dr. Wentz's intellect would often shine. In addition, if she saw a weakness, especially in a cocky senior male resident, she was able to use her intellect to make sure all knew who was in authority. Fortunately for us, she softened her approach with the medical students.

The competition for the first IVF baby was greatly increased because of Howard and Georgeanna Seegar Jones, IVF pioneers in Norfolk, Virginia. They had finished very successful academic careers and were enjoying retirement when they were encouraged to begin the Jones Institute, dedicated to performing the first successful IVF cycle in our country. They came out of retirement and formed an IVF team in Norfolk. And to make it even more interesting, Georgeanna Seegar Jones was Dr. Wentz's mentor, and the Joneses' son was a gynecologic cancer specialist at Vanderbilt, working alongside Dr. Wentz in the Ob/Gyn department. The connections were amazing. In 1981, the moon shot for the first IVF baby was on, and all the important personalities were prepared for the moment. To a young and naive medical student, it seemed like a competition to be the first, but in reality, all the important players had great love and respect for each other. It was actually a collaboration. It was fun being a medical student during this time, especially since I was strongly considering a career choice in IVF. The excitement was palpable, even during Dr. Wentz's team corrections during some of the early failures.

I will never forget the day during my third-year rotation when Dr. Jones (the son at Vanderbilt) proudly walked into the department and exclaimed, "My parents did it! They conceived the first IVF baby in America!" He was tall, in good shape, and carried himself with an air of confidence. Yet raised by genteel Southern academicians, he was respectful and courteous to a fault. He proclaimed the news in a way that brought quick cheers and celebration from the Vanderbilt team.

We were all excited because it was such an historic and world-changing moment. Dr. Wentz did not skip a beat and kept focused on the task at hand. Fortunately, Vanderbilt soon followed course. Dr. Wentz encouraged me along the way and even suggested that I consider an Ob/Gyn residency at the University of Connecticut under her friend and my next mentor, a renowned infertility expert named Dr. Dan Riddick.

During residency, my career path was settled as I was gently guided toward an infertility fellowship. When I started my fellowship in reproductive endocrinology and infertility at the University of Vermont, I was fully engulfed in the history and the future of this new field. It was an exciting time as people all over the country tried to begin IVF programs. Few specialists even knew how to do it. There were no businesses supporting IVF at that time, so we all had to make the media, purify the water, and come up with novel protocols for egg maturation. It's not easy starting with an egg in a dish and progressing to a baby at delivery.

I was a first-year fellow who knew very little, and Dr. Riddick, Chairman of the Ob/Gyn Department, and Dr. Mark Gibson, Fellowship Director of the Infertility Division, decided that I needed to learn IVF. Neither one of them felt fully comfortable in the new and emerging field. The University of Vermont had tried several cycles that were all unsuccessful. In addition, the field was rapidly changing since it was in its infancy. New medicines were being developed, and someone had just recently figured out how to perform an egg retrieval through the vagina. So they sent me, along with our lab director and nurse, to visit two programs, one in Nevada and one in Massachusetts. Both had experienced success. I learned all I could, wrote down everything everyone taught me, and brought it back to Vermont. As a first-year fellow with no authority and little knowledge, I navigated a total redo of the program and launched the new program in the winter of 1989 during the second year of my fellowship.

The IVF nurse in Vermont was a lot like me—very green, very excited, very confident, and yet very inexperienced in IVF. She was perfect for the job. Without any history and for no good reason, she quickly developed trust in me. She supported all my decisions as I changed everything from the medicine protocols to the equipment. Neither one of us had anyone else to confide in while at work, so it was a perfect partnership and friendship. The lab director was a classic intellectual and scientist. She was wonderful in the lab and knew the science of cell culture better than anyone else. However, she could not even begin to understand how the patients were handling all of this. The art of medicine was lost on her, yet her role was equally important to my role or the nurse's role. It was a very unusual team. But as in much of life, team unity was vital, and we functioned as a team at a very high level even though we really didn't know what we were doing.

As a fellow, I was not in charge. In everything, I answered to an attending physician. I knew instinctively that failure would fall squarely on their shoulders, not mine. But in the IVF program at Vermont, they trusted me to make all the big decisions. Looking back, I stand amazed at the faith and trust the leadership placed in me. They were perfect mentors, understanding who I was at my core and allowing my gifts to mature. At the same time, they knew what failure on my part would do to me, but they entrusted it to me anyway. It set the tone for both my career and my ability to handle tough situations and make difficult decisions. I will always be grateful to them for the confidence they demonstrated in me. Never underestimate the power of believing in those around you, especially if they are young and immature. A good mentor can totally change the path of a young mind. Everything can bend in the right direction with an appropriate mentor-mentee relationship.

In life, as with infertility, timing is critical. At our core, we desire to be encouraged and honored, even though we grow up in a world that often discourages and shames. The growth of maturity is not like a straight line through life but more like a mountain range with plenty of ups and downs. We all need a foundation of love and truth. But we also need valleys of adversity and peaks of success. Valleys and peaks without a strong foundation can wear us out too soon before our muscles are developed. A good foundation without any peaks or valleys leaves us wanting more, often setting our sights on lesser goals.

However, when there is a strong foundation followed by a moment of great success and honor, it can propel the immature soul into a place of confidence and faith, striving to accomplish more out of a sense of desire than a sense of need.

What does all this have to do with a young doctor in his third year of a fellowship at the University of Vermont? Let me tell you. The new IVF program at Vermont was successful that year. It was a great day. The weight on our shoulders had been lifted, and we were credited with the first IVF pregnancy in the state of Vermont, as well as one of the few successful programs in the country at that time. As I moved into my third year of fellowship, we grew the program and continued to experience success.

Our first pregnancy was due to be born in May at the end of my third year in fellowship. I was planning to leave Vermont in June and begin my career in North Carolina. One door was opening, and another was closing. I was very proud of my time at Vermont and settled into a position in the background as I planned my move to North Carolina. I helped get the next team ready. I was both proud of my accomplishments and yet nervous to do it all over again. My emotions were all over the place.

Based on this transitional season, I decided to use the time for knee surgery. I had injured my left knee while skiing in Vermont three years earlier. It was getting worse, so I had reconstructive knee surgery in May. Coincidentally, the C-section for Vermont's first IVF baby was scheduled the week after my surgery. While the news cameras would be there, I knew that the attention would be on the fellowship director since he was the head of the program and the one staying at Vermont. But those on the inside knew of my role, and of course, the patient knew.

Not wanting to take away from the event for the others on the team, I quietly maneuvered my wheelchair to the labor and delivery desk. My leg was in a cast, and I could not walk. I sat there patiently, waiting for the news of the first IVF birth in the program and the state. Let the attention go to the Vermont team. I was excited about my new career and would fade quietly into Vermont's history books.

As I was sitting there, a nurse came out of the delivery room and said, "The couple wants you in the room when the baby is born." I was shocked since I was not her doctor anymore and the surgery room was supposed to be a sterile environment. Before I could say, "That's impossible. I'm in a wheelchair," she grabbed the back of my chair and dragged me backward into the delivery room. Somewhat embarrassed, I tried to hide in the corner of the room, worried that the nurse had overstepped her authority. She might be fired for this, I thought.

As the baby emerged from the incision, there were spontaneous cheers around the room. Everyone knew the importance of the moment. All the doctors in the room were proud to be part of the first IVF baby in the state.

However, in the corner of the room was a young doctor who felt the proudest. There were plenty of congratulations to go around, but I knew what this experience had done to a fledgling fellow. I came to the Northeast as a small-town boy from Tennessee but was leaving a confident and different young man. This knowledge was settling into my heart in the corner of that delivery room, and I was fully content to let this be one of those special private moments that I pondered in my heart.

While the woman was being stitched up, the couple looked over at me, beaming as proud parents who had weathered the trials of infertility and put their faith in a young and inexperienced fellow, and said, "We're going to name our baby after you."

All the attention, all the news coverage, all the accolades faded into oblivion at that moment. A glow began to emerge from my soul, and I began to realize the depth of this honor. Money, gifts, and fame are nice, but they do not touch the significance of honor and encouragement to the human soul, especially during a critical time of development.

Never underestimate your ability to give encouragement. You just might light a fire in someone that becomes the engine for greater good. Trust your instincts regarding the timing of giving someone honor. If it's too early, they might not be ready for it. If it's too late, they might be discouraged and unable to be propelled by it. But given at just the right moment, it can set a young soul on fire. And don't assume that all gifts can be held or neatly wrapped up and handed to someone. Perhaps the best gift can only be held in the recesses of the human heart.

Dr. Deaton's Prescription: Encouragement is a gift that to be truly helpful must be given with truth and honesty. Vain flattery can do more damage than good, and sarcasm inflicts long-term pain. Giving encouragement must be practiced, but don't be afraid of failure. None of us are perfect encouragers.

My prescription for you is to find one person you can encourage, whether in a letter, a phone call, or in person. Then reflect on their response to your encouragement and how you felt offering it.

How will you follow this prescription?

UNDERSTANDING THE ROLE OF GENETICS ON YOUR JOURNEY

One of the most dynamic and exciting frontiers in IVF involves the field of genetics. From Watson and Crick's groundbreaking discovery of DNA's structure to the mapping of the human genome and the development of blood tests for genetic diagnoses, genetics is experiencing a remarkable renaissance. This rapid pace of change can understandably be confusing for both fertility specialists and patients alike. While the information in this chapter is current, it's important to recognize that this is a field that evolves quickly. Here's a summary of key genetic concepts relevant to IVF today.

Currently, there are three common genetic screening tests offered to individuals and couples navigating infertility.

Karyotype: This is a blood test that analyzes the number and structure of chromosomes in an individual, a fetus, or an embryo. Humans typically have 46 chromosomes arranged in 23 pairs. Women have two X chromosomes (46 XX), and men have one X and one Y chromosome (46 XY). Karyotyping is often performed on individuals with birth defects, fetuses with abnormalities detected during pregnancy, and couples experiencing recurrent miscarriages.

The majority of miscarriages are due to random chromosomal abnormalities in the fetus, with trisomy 16 (an extra 16th chromosome) being a common example. This risk of a random fetal chromosome anomaly greatly increases with older maternal age. While routine testing of miscarriage tissue isn't always recommended, it may be considered in cases of multiple pregnancy losses. If you have suffered multiple losses, you or your partner's own chromosomes may carry what is called a balanced translocation.

Thanks to recent advancements, we can now perform karyotyping on embryos before implantation, a process called pre-implantation genetic testing for aneuploidy (PGT-A), allowing for the use of euploid embryos with the correct number of chromosomes (46). An aneuploid embryo is one that does not have the normal 46 chromosomes. This technique increases the success rate of IVF and lowers the risk of miscarriages since embryos that ultimately miscarry have been screened out and not used.

Recessive Disease Screening: Many genetic diseases are recessive, which means they only manifest if an individual inherits two copies of the mutated gene, one from each parent. Carriers who possess only one copy of the gene are typically unaffected. That is why recessive diseases can appear unexpectedly in families. Once a child is diagnosed with a recessive condition, the parents are usually tested to identify if they are carriers. If both parents are carriers of the same recessive gene, each pregnancy has a 25% chance of the embryo inheriting two copies and developing the disease, a 50% chance of the embryo being a carrier (like the parents), and a 25% chance of the embryo inheriting two normal copies. Most fertility clinics offer recessive disease screening to one or both partners. If one partner is found to be a carrier of a recessive gene, the other partner is then tested for the same gene. It's important to note that most people carry at least one recessive gene; the key is whether both partners carry the same recessive gene. Sperm and egg donors undergo automatic and comprehensive recessive disease screening. Current technology allows screening for hundreds of recessive diseases, and this number continues to expand.

Dominant Genetic Disease Screening: In contrast to recessive conditions, dominant genetic diseases manifest when an individual inherits only one copy of the mutated gene. These conditions typically don't "hide" in families but are seen passing from an affected parent to approximately half of their children. This 50% inheritance rate occurs because during reproduction a parent contributes only one chromosome from each pair to their offspring. If a parent carries a dominant gene, there is a 50% chance that the child will inherit that chromosome with the affected gene. Examples of dominant genes include the BRCA genes associated with increased breast cancer risk, some forms of polycystic kidney disease, and Huntington's disease, a debilitating neurological disorder.

If there's a dominant condition in your family history or if you and your partner are at risk of having a child with a recessive disease (because you are both carriers of the same gene), current technology allows for testing not only yourselves but also your embryos. This is called pre-implantation genetic testing for monogenic diseases (PGT-M).

Therefore, during your initial consultation with your fertility specialist, a basic karyotype is generally not needed unless there's a history of recurrent miscarriages. However, most couples opt for recessive carrier screening for one or both partners. Testing for dominant genes relies on a thorough family history, so it's helpful to come prepared with information about any significant inherited conditions in your family.

Often, a crucial decision regarding genetic testing needs to be made before starting your IVF cycle. Your provider will discuss this early on to allow ample time for consideration.

Even in the absence of known recessive or dominant genes of concern, many patients choose to undergo PGT-A to screen their embryos for missing or extra chromosomes. This can potentially increase the success rate of IVF, lower the risk of miscarriage, and reduce the chance of a child with certain chromosomal abnormalities. PGT-A is strongly recommended for women over the age of 35 as the incidence of chromosomal errors in embryos rises significantly after that age. If you decide to proceed with PGT (either PGT-A or PGT-M), your embryos will be biopsied at the blastocyst stage. That involves creating a small opening in the embryo's outer shell (zona pellucida) and carefully removing approximately five to six cells from the trophectoderm (the layer that will become the placenta), thus not harming the cells that will form the baby. All biopsied embryos are then frozen, and the genetic testing results for each embryo typically take 10 to 14 days. Your clinic will schedule a consultation to discuss the results, and a frozen embryo transfer will be planned for the following month, assuming you have at least one euploid (46 XX or 46 XY) blastocyst.

A final note: I have also worked with many couples who choose to give every embryo a chance regardless of PGT-A results. While fertility specialists would not generally transfer aneuploid embryos with conditions incompatible with life (found in the majority of abnormal embryos), the decision regarding the transfer of aneuploid embryos that can result in a live birth can be very complex for some couples. Examples include Turner syndrome (missing an X chromosome) and trisomy 21 (an extra 21st chromosome). There are also various partial trisomies that may be detected by PGT-A. Children born with these conditions may be affected but can lead fulfilling and meaningful lives.

If you are considering transferring all embryos that are compatible with life, it's important to be prepared for potentially difficult decisions during pregnancy and after birth. The ethical considerations surrounding PGT can be challenging, and fertility providers want you to be well-informed before making these decisions. Don't hesitate to discuss your values and beliefs with your doctor or consider scheduling a consultation with a genetic counselor. Most fertility offices have genetic counselors available who can provide valuable information and support before you need to make these important choices.

CHAPTER 9

IT IS OFTEN DARKEST JUST BEFORE THE DAWN

S he was delightful at her first visit and very engaging, talkative, and obviously in love with her husband. She was very small with jet black hair, barely weighing 100 pounds yet always in control of the room. She would openly fight with her husband, especially when he made an innocent comment trying to minimize the pain she was feeling. But he always fought back. It appeared to be a wonderful marriage, one with mutual respect and love.

She joked about how much she hated needles, fully understanding that her infertility journey would probably involve lots and lots of needles. I told her she would become a pro at getting blood drawn and giving herself shots. I knew her chances were high and that I would be sending her back pregnant to her obstetrician in no time. After failing some simpler treatments, they decided to move aggressively to IVF.

They were fortunate to have full insurance coverage, so there would not be a financial burden—just all those needles.

There was also another stress they carried. They were both part of a culture that puts incredible pressure on adult children to produce grandchildren. In my family and in many American families, we are more willing to embrace a couple without children. It's not always easy for the extended family. Subtle hints and comments may come, but at the end of the day, they support their children. But in her culture, the culture her parents were born into and passed on to her, the pressure is intense. And my patient's parents had flown to America to support their daughter and her husband in this process. Everyone was involved in her cycle; all eyes were on her unfolding journey. If I was unsuccessful, I knew there would be a lot of people I would need to answer to.

They embarked on their IVF journey with the creation of several embryos, some that were frozen and two that were placed into her uterus. And as I expected, she was pregnant eight days later. The couple was elated, told everyone in their family, and were referred back to their obstetrician.

But something went wrong with the pregnancy, and she lost her child at a very late stage of her pregnancy. The emotions went from the highest high to the lowest low. Grieving is healthy, and she grieved appropriately. Counseling was needed. But the feelings of inadequacy, guilt, and helplessness persisted. Her husband was very supportive, and often the bright spots in our times together were when the husband and wife argued about next steps or feelings. They were very good together. His weaknesses were balanced by her strengths, and her weaknesses were balanced by his strengths. But the visits were intense, and I would often switch from infertility doctor to marriage counselor.

After a long time, they came back and tried their frozen embryos. None worked. Now the feelings surrounding the loss were combined with the feelings of getting older, and the sessions became more intense. After more waiting and against my advice to consider adoption or donor eggs, they came back for another IVF cycle. The first time we did this felt easy with lots of optimism and hope. Now, after the miscarriage and failed embryo transfers, this one felt almost hopeless. A loss of hope and depression are often the case with greater pressure on each attempt.

In order to lower the chance of a miscarriage or a genetic defect, we decided to perform genetic testing on the embryos. While normal in today's world of IVF, this was not commonly done at the time but seemed the perfect solution for this couple. We would transfer only genetically normal embryos, thereby increasing the chance of success and minimizing the chance of a pregnancy loss. Embryos with too few or too many chromosomes don't implant or lead to a miscarriage. This couple had gone through enough, so I decided to optimize their chances. Despite our best efforts, we got only a few embryos, and only one was genetically normal. It didn't work. There was more grief, feelings of failure, and pressure from the parents.

I felt like I was making their situation worse. If their marriage didn't survive, their infertility treatments would be high on the list of causes.

They came back for another talk. The emotions seemed to be getting worse, and the marriage counseling seemed to be increasing. The pressure to be pregnant was intense, so they would not consider adoption or living as a couple without children. I knew in my heart they could become a happy and content couple even without children, but they would hear none of this. They had to have a good pregnancy.

I encouraged them to consider donor eggs due to her age, and they agreed. Due to their culture, finding the right donor was difficult, but they persevered and found a perfect match for them. The donor was young, in her 20s, and should give high-quality eggs. Donor egg cycles, especially with the transfer of young embryos into a healthy uterus, have extremely high success rates, so I knew this would work. I took them from the depths of despair to a place of hope.

Hope is the best motivator in life. I never try to leave a couple with less hope than they came in with. Without hope, life can be difficult and tedious. Without hope, the tough times can become unbearable, and we all have tough times. When we pillow our heads at night in a season of adversity, it's hope that gets us up in the morning—hope for a better life, hope for healthy relationships, hope for children.

Once again, to avoid any chance of a genetic defect in their child, we decided to perform genetic testing on the embryos created from the donor eggs and her husband's sperm. I would not normally recommend this because donors are all young and don't tend to make many genetically abnormal embryos. But this was not a normal couple. The donor came to our institution, and I retrieved a bunch of eggs. We created 10 high-quality embryos and tested all of them. Much to our delight, we had seven genetically normal embryos.

After years and years of frustration, emotions, and marriage counseling, we were near the end. It was hard to imagine this not working. In fact, each embryo had a roughly 70% chance of implanting and leading to a successful pregnancy. Miscarriages and pregnancy complications were greatly reduced since these were genetically normal embryos. Often at their visits, I had to fight her statements of "being cursed." I tried to maintain my optimism with these seven normal embryos from a young donor, but it was hard. It seemed like the couple was putting a large fence around their hearts, trying not to let hope in. And yet this had to work. There are times to be guarded, and there are times to be full of hope. This was a time to repair their broken hearts and bring hope and stability back into their lives.

After three embryo transfers, all genetically normal, we still had no success. What were the odds? I began to question myself. Was I missing something? Was her uterus not able to carry a pregnancy? And yet she had carried her first pregnancy far into the second trimester. I am accustomed to patients losing hope, but most of the time, I bring hope back in. And yet now, I was losing hope and fearing that I was making their lives worse.

I often hear patients say, "I must be cursed" or "I am being punished" or "I don't measure up to other women" or "I'm not blessed." And always, I am the one who refutes all those statements. But now, with this couple, I felt myself starting to question some of my foundational beliefs. There was no scientific reason why they should have had all these failures. The numbers did not add up. There must be something else going on that I was missing. Couples come to me for help, but now I was trying to find someone to help me.

After her third failure with genetically normal donor embryos and now having only four left, I was determined to leave no stone unturned. Therefore, my only option was surrogacy—finding another woman who could carry these embryos. Even though I had no good reason to suggest this route, I did not want to use up all her embryos without success. Surrogacy is complicated both legally and ethically, and yet I was willing to put them through this because the implications of failure were too hard even for me to accept.

This couple was in too deep to get out, so the only option was to go deeper. I suggested surrogacy. The tears flowed. Every time we met, I tried to bring it up. The tears flowed. Finally, one day she was on the schedule for an ultrasound to get ready for her cycle. I had a visiting nurse with me that day, so we walked in the room, and I introduced the two women to each other.

Since we were planning her cycle, I once again brought up the concept of considering surrogacy before we ran out of embryos. Furthermore, I had noticed that on all her recent visits, her husband was no longer with her. They were still together—just unable to bear this burden as a couple any longer. I began to fear for her marriage and her life.

Before all the words came out of my mouth, she wailed, "Dr. Deaton, you have to get me pregnant!" It was then I realized

I had become too emotionally wrapped up in her success, so I backed off, committed to never mentioning surrogacy again. While I can lay out all the options, the couple needs to make the final decision.

There are times when a doctor doesn't know what to say to a patient. Even with lots of experience, having walked through every possible situation, the pain can be so great that I often don't know what to say. Words can be cheap. People most need to know that I'm there and that I'm rooting for them.

We proceeded with her cycle and transferred a normal female embryo. Nine months later, we all celebrated greatly at the little girl's birth. No one will ever explain to me why that cycle worked while the countless others ended in heartache. But when she asked me after the delivery what I thought about her journey, I looked at her precious daughter and said, "If it weren't for all the countless losses and heartache, you wouldn't be holding this girl. So cherish her. Your journey has been all about your daughter."

Their journey could have taken any direction—despair, breakup, giving up, or unsurpassed joy. They chose their path and came to realize that it is darkest just before the dawn. But what an incredible sunrise they were able to share. At times it is appropriate to ponder where you are and make a significant change in life. At other times it is necessary to hang in there, persevere, and not give up on your dreams. Only you can determine the path. Don't be afraid to seek help as you navigate the emotional roller coaster of life.

Dr. Deaton's Prescription: Hope is the greatest ally you have in caring for your health. If a patient comes to see me who has lost all hope and has given up, it can limit what I can do medically or scientifically to help that person. What you believe about yourself and your future greatly affects how you will respond to medicine and clinical treatment.

Today I want you to do a checkup on your hope. Do you still have hope for the things you long for? Don't try to figure out how these things will come about. Leave that for someone else. You need to continue to hold onto hope and trust that there is someone who cares for you more than you can possibly imagine.

How will you follow this prescription?

THE SCIENCE BEHIND IVF: A STEP-BY-STEP GUIDE

How does IVF actually work? Think of it as a carefully orchestrated process where fertility specialists guide and control your menstrual cycle to facilitate egg retrieval and embryo transfer. While every individual and couple is unique, the fundamental steps followed by most fertility providers are outlined in order below.

Ovarian Suppression: Remember FSH, the hormone that stimulates the development of antral follicles into dominant follicles? Naturally, FSH levels rise early in your cycle. However, in IVF, we aim for the development of multiple eggs simultaneously. To prevent a premature rise in FSH that could lead to the early development of only one egg, most clinics utilize a short course of oral contraceptives to suppress your natural cycle. While this is the most common approach, another method involves placing an estrogen patch approximately 7–10 days after ovulation, which also suppresses FSH. However, that requires precise ovulation tracking and can be more complex if ovulation is uncertain.

The suppression of FSH is not mandatory, and there are two other methods employed by some programs. First, it is also possible to simply start the ovarian stimulation with your period. Second, in time-sensitive situations such as for cancer patients, stimulation may begin during any phase of the cycle since early antral follicles are always present and ready to grow.

Baseline Assessment: Before your ovarian stimulation begins, often a few days after the last oral contraceptive pill, you'll typically undergo a transvaginal ultrasound to ensure your ovaries are at a baseline, which means they are suppressed and free of cysts. If this is confirmed, you're ready to begin the ovarian stimulation phase.

Ovarian Stimulation: As mentioned earlier, FSH is the key hormone that stimulates your ovaries to grow follicles, each containing an immature egg. If your baseline ultrasound is clear, you'll begin daily FSH injections. They come in two main forms: recombinant pure FSH and urinary-derived FSH that also contains some LH. Many fertility specialists prefer including a small amount of LH in their stimulation protocols. The FSH dosage is carefully determined and often guided by your AMH level. The goal is to stimulate the development of a good number of eggs without causing an excessive response, which can lead to a potentially dangerous condition called ovarian hyperstimulation syndrome (OHSS).

- *Low AMH (typically under 2.5):* In these cases, the highest starting dose of FSH is often used, as the risk of OHSS is very low.
- *High AMH:* A lower starting dose is often preferred to grow a sufficient number of eggs while minimizing the risk of OHSS.

Other factors such as body mass index, age, and previous responses to these medications also influence the starting dose.

Monitoring: Once you begin FSH injections, you'll have regular office visits every two to three days for both a transvaginal ultrasound to monitor follicle growth and blood tests to track your estrogen, progesterone, and LH levels. Based on your individual response, the FSH dosage may be adjusted up or down to optimize egg development while minimizing the risk of OHSS.

Trigger Shot: After approximately 8–12 days of FSH injections and monitoring, your cohort of dominant follicles will typically be ready for egg retrieval. However, the eggs within these follicles are still immature and require an LH surge to reach final maturation. This final step of the stimulation process involves a trigger shot administered on the last day of stimulation. There are two main ways to mimic the natural LH surge and trigger egg maturation.

- *Human Chorionic Gonadotropin (hCG) Injection:* hCG is the same hormone produced during pregnancy and detected in pregnancy tests. Importantly for IVF, hCG binds to LH receptors and acts similarly to LH, thus causing egg maturation.

- *Gonadotropin-Releasing Hormone (GnRH) Agonist Injection:* This medication stimulates your pituitary gland to release a significant surge of your own LH, thus triggering egg maturation. The choice between these two trigger methods often depends on the risk of OHSS. hCG can exacerbate OHSS if a large number of eggs have developed. In such cases, a GnRH agonist trigger is often preferred as it carries a lower risk of OHSS. Some clinics may make the decision based on the individual patient's response, while others may predominantly use GnRH agonists to minimize OHSS risk. In some situations, a combination of both (co-trigger) may be used. Regardless of the method, the timing of the trigger shot is critical as eggs will begin to release from your ovaries approximately 38–40 hours later.

Egg Retrieval: The trigger shot is given in the evening, and the egg retrieval procedure is scheduled for the morning approximately 35–36 hours later. For this procedure you will be under heavy sedation usually administered by an anesthesia provider, ensuring you feel little or no pain. The retrieval is performed transvaginally using an ultrasound probe with a needle guide attached. Your provider will visualize the follicles on the ultrasound and guide a needle through the top of the vagina directly into each follicle. The follicular fluid is then drained, and in most cases the mature eggs are found in this fluid. Draining all the follicles usually takes between 10 and 30 minutes, depending on the number of follicles. Afterward, you'll recover in a designated area, and most women wake up quickly and are able to leave within an hour. While you won't experience pain during the procedure, you may have some cramping and discomfort later in the day, which is usually well-managed with over-the-counter pain relievers such as acetaminophen or ibuprofen. In cases of OHSS, discomfort may persist for several days. You will need someone to drive you home, but many women feel well enough to take a walk or have a light dinner later that day. Be sure to discuss any specific limitations with your provider.

Egg Identification and Incubation: The aspirated follicular fluid is immediately passed to the embryology lab, often through a window connected to the retrieval room. The embryologist meticulously identifies the eggs and places them in a specialized incubator. The eggs remain in the incubator for approximately three to four hours before fertilization is attempted. During that time, they are examined for maturity (specifically the presence of a polar body, a small cellular structure indicating maturity). The majority of retrieved eggs are typically mature and suitable for fertilization. Cases of low egg maturity can be very frustrating, but techniques can be employed by your IVF team to lessen this chance in future cycles.

Sperm Preparation and Fertilization: A sperm sample is necessary for fertilization. Unless you are using previously frozen sperm (donor sperm or a testicular sample), your partner will need to provide a fresh sample on the day of retrieval. That can be arranged to ensure comfort and privacy. Many men provide their sample while their partner is undergoing the egg retrieval. Others may bring a previously collected sample with them. Discuss the most convenient option with your provider. After the eggs have incubated for three to four hours, they are removed and fertilized using one of two methods. The majority of couples undergo intracytoplasmic sperm injection (ICSI) where a single sperm is directly injected into each mature egg. ICSI is the standard procedure for male factor infertility (which accounts for about half of all cases) and is also frequently used in unexplained infertility or when only a small number of eggs are retrieved. If the sperm quality is excellent, the embryologist may opt for conventional insemination where thousands of sperm are placed near each egg to allow natural fertilization. Trust your embryology lab to choose the optimal method, but feel free to discuss any preferences or concerns with your provider. IVF providers designate the egg retrieval or fertilization day as Day 0.

Fertilization Check (Day 1): Approximately 18–22 hours after fertilization (the following morning), the embryology lab performs a fertilization check. They examine each egg for the presence of two pronuclei—one representing the egg's nucleus and the other the sperm's nucleus. The presence of two pronuclei confirms successful fertilization. Shortly after this time, the two pronuclei will fuse into a single nucleus.

Embryo Development (Days 2–6): Following the fertilization check, the embryos are left undisturbed to develop in the incubator. Most IVF programs allow the fertilized eggs to develop for 4–6 days, reaching the blastocyst stage. A blastocyst is a more advanced embryo containing 100–120 cells. It's important to remember that there is natural attrition in human reproduction. Not all mature eggs will fertilize, and only about 40%–50% of fertilized eggs will develop into usable, high-quality blastocysts. Therefore, don't expect every retrieved egg to become a baby. For a woman under 35, roughly seven retrieved eggs may lead to one live birth. This highlights the importance of AMH as an indicator of potential egg yield. Retrieving only a few eggs may unfortunately mean no viable embryos in that cycle. The blastocyst contains a fluid-filled cavity, an outer shell called the zona pellucida, and these two distinct cell types:

- *Inner Cell Mass:* These cells will eventually develop into a baby.
- *Trophectoderm:* These cells will form the placenta and membranes.

Pre-Implantation Genetic Testing (PGT) (Optional): Often, a crucial decision at the blastocyst stage involves PGT, which is commonly offered to couples undergoing IVF. Briefly, PGT is typically performed at the blastocyst stage and involves carefully removing 5–6 cells from the trophectoderm (the outer layer that becomes the placenta), thus not harming the inner cell mass that develops into the baby. Two main types of PGT are relevant for this discussion:

- *PGT-A (Aneuploidy Screening):* This is essentially a chromosome count of the embryo, aiming for the normal number of 46. Most embryo implantation failures and miscarriages are due to aneuploidy (missing or extra chromosomes). The incidence of aneuploidy in embryos increases significantly with maternal age over 35.
- *PGT-M (Monogenic Disease Testing):* If you and your partner carry the same recessive gene or if one of you carries a dominant gene for a specific inherited condition, specialized genetic probes can be created to test your embryos for these conditions. Both PGT-A and PGT-M require coordination with a genetic testing center and can add costs that are often not covered by insurance.

Embryo Transfer (Fresh vs. Frozen): If you opt not to undergo PGT, you may be a candidate for a fresh embryo transfer where a blastocyst is placed into your uterus approximately five days after egg retrieval. However, fresh transfers are not always the best option, particularly for the following:

- Patients undergoing PGT since the test results are not available in time for a fresh transfer.
- Patients with a high progesterone level on the day of the trigger shot since this can desynchronize the uterine lining and make it less receptive to the embryo.

- Patients with high estrogen levels and a high risk of OHSS. A successful fresh transfer in these cases significantly increases the risk of developing severe OHSS, and there is evidence that high estrogen levels may make the uterus less receptive to the blastocyst.

Frozen Embryo Transfer (FET): If a fresh transfer is not recommended or if you have embryos that have undergone PGT, you will proceed with a frozen embryo transfer (FET) cycle. In an FET cycle, your uterus is carefully prepared to be receptive to the thawed blastocyst. The following two main methods are used to prepare the uterine lining:

- *Programmed Cycle:* This involves administering high-dose estrogen for about two weeks followed by a transvaginal ultrasound to assess the endometrial thickness and appearance (ideally a trilayer pattern). Since estrogen typically suppresses ovarian activity, your ovaries remain quiet. Once the endometrium is adequately thickened, you'll begin progesterone supplementation. The embryo transfer is typically scheduled for 5–7 days after starting progesterone as this is generally the window of optimal uterine receptivity. Progesterone can be administered via intramuscular injections or vaginal preparations.

- *Natural or Modified Natural Cycle FET:* In this approach you are allowed to develop an egg naturally or with the help of a mild fertility drug. You'll have a mid-cycle ultrasound to monitor follicle development. If the follicle grows, hormone levels are appropriate, and the endometrium is adequately thickened and trilayered, you'll likely receive a trigger shot to stimulate ovulation and progesterone production. The FET will be scheduled for seven days after the trigger shot. This method is more natural and allows the ovary to produce its own hormones.

Studies suggest that success rates for the first FET are similar between programmed and natural cycles. However, if the first FET is unsuccessful, your provider may discuss using the alternative protocol for subsequent attempts. While IVF providers typically place the blastocyst on the sixth day of progesterone exposure, there is some controversial evidence that a few women are more receptive to the embryo on the fifth or seventh day of progesterone exposure. If you have failed embryo transfers, you may want to discuss this with your provider. Finally, there is also emerging evidence that endometriosis patients who fail transfers may benefit from an alternative protocol that suppresses the endometriosis tissue. Again, discuss this with your provider if you have failed transfers.

Pre-Transfer Discussion: Before the actual transfer, it is important to discuss a few key factors with your provider, particularly the number of embryos to transfer. With current technology, especially after PGT, transferring only one embryo is strongly recommended to minimize the risk of multiple pregnancies (twins or triplets), which carry significant risks for both the mother and the babies. If you underwent PGT-A and know the gender of your embryos, your clinic may allow you to choose the gender to transfer. On the day of the transfer, you'll typically arrive with a full bladder. A full bladder is needed in order to see the transfer catheter on the ultrasound as it enters your uterine cavity. Also, many women have an anterior curve from the cervix into the uterus, and the full bladder can straighten out the uterus and make the transfer easier for the provider. Typically, you will have a meeting with your partner (if applicable), your fertility specialist, and an embryologist to review the embryos, confirm which one will be transferred, and sign any necessary consent forms.

Embryo Transfer Procedure: The FET is usually an emotionally significant moment, one you have been expecting for quite a long time. Fertility providers strive to make this a positive experience for you and your partner. The transfer is performed using a very thin, soft catheter that is gently guided into your uterus under real-time ultrasound visualization. While you won't be able to see the actual embryo, you can observe the catheter's placement. This is an important time to ask any remaining questions. The transfer is usually painless, although you might feel a sensation as the catheter passes through your cervix. A full bladder can also cause some discomfort. Once the transfer is complete and you're allowed to get up, you can generally resume most normal activities. Despite common anxieties, the embryo will not "fall out." If this were the case, natural pregnancies would be impossible. Try to relax and be patient during the 8–10 day wait for your pregnancy test. There is nothing you can do to influence the outcome at this point, so try to avoid excessive worry. Discuss strategies for managing the waiting period with your provider.

Embryo Storage: Hopefully, you will have additional high-quality embryos that can be cryopreserved (frozen) for potential future pregnancies. These embryos will remain frozen until you and your partner decide their fate. Most IVF programs will discuss the various options with you prior to or during your cycle. While most couples retain their embryos for later use, other options include discarding, donating for scientific research, or donating to another couple. This can be a complex and personal decision that you and your partner should discuss openly. You will also need to decide before the process what happens to your embryos if one of you becomes incapacitated or you get divorced. These can be difficult decisions, so reach out to a trusted individual or counselor if you need help.

While the IVF process may seem overwhelming as you read through these steps, please try not to be anxious. Your IVF clinic will have dedicated team members, often IVF nurses, who are specifically trained to guide you through every stage. They are there to support you, so don't hesitate to ask any questions that arise. The doctors, nurses, and support staff are all committed to helping you achieve your goal of building your family. They are on your side even if you feel alone at times.

CHAPTER 10

KEEPING THE MAIN THING THE MAIN THING

It was very early in my career when I was much younger. After medical school, an Ob/Gyn residency, and finally a fellowship in reproductive endocrinology and infertility, I felt well-trained and ready to begin my career. My upbringing also blended nicely with my chosen profession in gynecology. I watched my mom forge a career as a working mother in the 1960s and 1970s. She was independent and strong yet a working woman without an advanced degree in a time ruled by men. If she had been born a little later, I'm sure she would have run a company.

Furthermore, my older sister, Jan, was a significant influence in my early life. She would come home from her first-grade classes, sit me down, and teach me what she had learned, especially math. I learned at an early age not to say no to her. Through her, I developed a love of education and a love of science. I was able to watch her navigate a man's world, rising quickly in her company to a place of authority. I also watched her struggle after the birth of her first child. Would she continue her career? In those days, it was complicated for a woman to climb the ladder of success while raising a family. These unique struggles that women faced back then continue to this day. I came to understand these struggles at a young age. I'll always be thankful to my mom and sister for teaching me the value of women, both at home and in the workplace.

So with a passion and foundation for women's issues and 11 years of training, I knew how to do my job. Or did I? A couple early in my career taught me a valuable lesson, one that was overlooked in all my training.

Dino and Leigh were a very typical couple—I would even say a stereotypical infertility couple. They were in their mid-30s, professional, and well-prepared to accept a child into their lives. Dino ran an important business in our town, and Leigh was a successful businesswoman. Friendly and outgoing, they were the type of couple everyone wanted to be around. They were financially secure and lived a full life. Now it was time to become parents. No hesitation. After all, it was the right thing to do. It was expected. To do anything else would be, well, odd. But it wasn't happening, so they came to see me.

We met for about 45 minutes, and I laid out a plan of attack. After all, I knew how to get people pregnant. I had all the tools at my disposal—excellent training, a faculty appointment at Wake Forest University School of Medicine, and a brand-new IVF program with all the bells and whistles. In the course of the workup, I determined that Leigh had diminished ovarian reserve, or poor egg quality. In other words, her ovaries were acting like they were near menopause. While I knew this would be difficult for them to hear, I was already planning a donor egg cycle in my mind that would have a high chance of success. I knew her uterus could carry a pregnancy; all she needed was an egg donor. I knew how to get them pregnant, and surely they would follow me down that path. After all, it was the right thing to do, and I was the bright and well-trained new doctor in town.

I called Dino and Leigh. As is my practice, I gave them a brief summary of the information on the phone and tried to lessen the blow. I suggested they come to my office for a talk to fully explore all their options. Of course, there were many options to consider such as IVF using Leigh's eggs, a donor egg cycle using her sister's eggs, or adoption.

Having had this discussion with other couples while I was in my training, I knew what to expect. The face-to-face visit would be difficult. Everyone wants a biological offspring, so they would need space and time to grieve this news. But with skills learned in training and honed in practice, I was sure I could lead them down a journey of either donor eggs or adoption. I knew the visit would be very emotional, possibly long, and fraught with danger. They might be upset, grieve, and then move on, or it could lead Leigh into a state of depression and anger. It could go either direction.

My nurse put them in my office and handed me the chart. I walked up to the door, took a deep breath, and rehearsed in my mind how I was going to handle this. But when I threw open the door, I came upon a scene that still makes me laugh. There was Leigh, sitting in Dino's lap, and they were making out like two high school kids in the back seat of a car.

Patients don't tend to make out while waiting for the doctor. And besides, if I had waited much longer, they could have actually been trying to get pregnant in my office! Furthermore, they were supposed to be devastated, grieving over the loss of a biological child. I've worked with thousands of couples and thus knew how difficult this journey would be for them. Yet they seemed different than most couples. So Dino, Leigh, and I gathered ourselves and began the conversation that taught me much about how to lead a well-lived life.

You see, Dino and Leigh kept the main thing the main thing. They didn't get married to have children; they got married because they were in love. Of course they wanted children, but they wanted each other more. Of course they would grieve not having children, but they would celebrate their love for each other even more. Of course, they had prepared themselves for all the changes that would come with a child, but they were fully committed to planning their journey as a couple, together. We talked, and I quickly realized in my heart that they would be fine as a child-free couple. Using her sister's eggs did not work for them, so I spoke about anonymous donor eggs and adoption. But they were content to enjoy the fullness of life as Dino and Leigh, a full family of two.

A person's happiness and contentment often hinge on the presence or absence of a certain blessing. Some men say, "I can't be content unless I get that job" or "I can't be happy unless I win that sports championship." Many couples in my office inwardly say, "We can't be content and complete unless we have a baby." But let's be honest. That type of thinking turns something good—a blessing—into an idol. Before long, you begin to line up your entire life around the one thing you're missing. All the good in your life seems gone, and your one desire takes over your life, often in a very bad way.

If your idol is having a baby, all other dreams take second place. Without thinking about it, patients often delay taking a new job, buying a new house, or going on a dream trip. They think, "How can we plan a move when we might get pregnant?" or "What if we plan a trip and then get pregnant and have to cancel?" The "what if" scenarios are endless. They also choose to keep their infertility a secret because they don't want to enter into discussions about their failures. Keeping a secret is hard, leading to a life of isolation. When isolated, we get out of balance. And when out of balance, we can fall.

Furthermore, if you're not careful, the absence of your chosen blessing can turn you into someone who feels unblessed or, worse, a victim. Your life begins to take a downward spiral since you begin to believe you have nothing. And believing a lie about yourself can change everything for the worse.

Thankfully, Dino and Leigh knew they were fortunate and lived their life out of fullness. I could imagine them saying, "We are so happy, and our love is overflowing, so we want to bring a child into the world to share that love. If we can't have a child, we'll grieve but continue life knowing how lucky and blessed we are." They didn't need a child to be complete; they wanted a child because they *were* complete.

I kept up with Dino and Leigh through her mother, a precious woman in our community. While I'm sure there were times they thought about a child, I believe they became the best aunt, uncle, friend, daughter, and son in the city. They were determined to live a full life, loving those around them with a depth that only increased once they opened their hearts to new possibilities. I've seen too many infertility couples put a wall around their hearts, not allowing the love of others in and not allowing themselves to celebrate the joy in their friends' lives that comes from having children. Infertility turns some inward, which can lead them into a life of guardedness where they are unwilling to enter into true relationship and the celebrations of others.

Dino and Leigh are a refreshing exception. With time and appropriate grieving, they have become content and continue to celebrate life, which is often defined by celebrating others. Many people value their love, and they are willing to give it. Even in their own disappointments, their hearts remain open and vulnerable, able to pour out and receive love. Their lives are full, and they are unwilling to diminish their lives because of a loss.

If you're on a journey of infertility, I hope it has a successful and happy resolution. Go see someone who is well-trained and compassionate to help you. You may encounter a young physician just starting out. If you do, teach them that the job is not only helping people get pregnant but also locking arms with the infertile couple on their journey and guiding them to their place of contentment, whether it is with a pregnancy, an adoption, or child-free living.

No two families look alike. Open your heart to all the possibilities. Grieve when needed, but don't forget the blessings all around you. Don't neglect or abandon your first love in a quest for another.

Dr. Deaton's Prescription: Often during a difficult time of soul-searching and introspection, your outward life can look unfamiliar, not only to yourself but also to those around you. We can easily forget to enjoy life when we feel the weight of the world on our shoulders. There's a tendency to retreat into our shell and simply wait for the storm to pass. But what if the storm lasts a long time? And what if, during our season of retreat, we become a different person and our relationships all change? You might emerge into a time of calm and blue skies but lonelier than before the storm hit. When facing a trial, go down the road most traveled and keep living life. You will emerge into a place of deeper joy and even deeper relationships.

Think about your greatest pursuit at this time in your life, perhaps one that is uniquely difficult to achieve. Is the pursuit becoming a strain on you? Is there another love of your life that is being pushed out by this pursuit? Are you losing your core values or other blessings in your life due to this pursuit?

Think about something important in your life that you have taken for granted, perhaps something that was a passion in an earlier season of your life. It can be a person, a hobby, or even an earlier interest of yours.

Go rekindle that flame.

How will you follow this prescription?

SHOULD YOU CONSIDER GOING STRAIGHT TO IVF?

In vitro fertilization stands as one of the monumental achievements of the 20th century. Since the birth of the first IVF baby in 1978, it was clear that this scientific breakthrough would revolutionize the field of infertility and have a profound impact globally. In the United States, the percentage of babies born via IVF has risen from 0% in 1980 to approximately 2.5% in 2024—about one in every 40 babies is conceived through IVF. In countries with universal insurance coverage for fertility treatments, this percentage is even higher, around 5%–10%. As advancements in genetics and egg development continue, this number is likely to keep increasing.

Given the high success rates of IVF and the markedly lower success rates of other treatments, some infertility specialists may readily recommend IVF as a first-line treatment. Don't interpret this advice as an aggressive, greedy doctor but rather as simple advice in helping you best get to your desired goal. However, it's crucial to exercise caution. While IVF is indeed the most appropriate option for certain couples, many others can achieve pregnancy with less intensive and less costly approaches. To help you navigate this critical decision, here are examples of specific situations where moving directly to IVF may be the most cost-effective and appropriate path.

- *Severe Male Factor Infertility:* While there isn't a universal definition, a "severe male factor" often involves a very low total motile count (TMC) in the semen analysis. If the TMC is under 5 million motile sperm, proceeding directly to IVF—often in conjunction with consultation with a male factor infertility specialist—is frequently recommended and often represents your best option.

- *Tubal Disease or Pelvic Scar Tissue:* Blocked fallopian tubes or significant pelvic scar tissue, often diagnosed through a patient's history (ectopic pregnancies, sexually transmitted infections, prior pelvic surgeries), can necessitate moving directly to IVF as other treatments are significantly less likely to be successful.

- *Low AMH:* If your AMH is low, time may not be on your side, especially if you want more than one child. While IVF can be expensive, if you delay pursuing IVF with a low AMH, you may significantly reduce your chances of conceiving with your own eggs. While purchasing donor eggs is always an option in this situation, most couples prioritize genetic continuity with their child. There isn't a specific AMH level threshold that dictates an immediate move to IVF, so this is a crucial conversation to have with your fertility doctor. This is especially true if you are considering banking embryos for future children.

- *Desire for Embryo Genetic Testing:* PGT offers the ability to biopsy an embryo and test either the total number of chromosomes (PGT-A) or for a specific inherited genetic disorder (PGT-M). There are three main reasons why you might consider IVF with PGT as a first line treatment.

  » *Known Inherited Genetic Disease:* If you or your partner carry a dominant gene (where a 50% chance of passing it on exists) or if both partners carry the same recessive gene (giving a 25% chance of the child being affected, such as with cystic fibrosis or sickle cell anemia), PGT-M can test embryos to identify those that are unaffected, which can then be placed into your uterus.

» *Increased Maternal Age (Over 35):* Women over 35 have a higher risk of having children with certain chromosomal abnormalities such as trisomy 21. PGT-A screens embryos for the correct number of chromosomes, called an euploid embryo. Abnormal embryos (aneuploid, with missing or extra chromosomes) often fail to implant or result in early miscarriage. Many older women opt for PGT-A to reduce the risk of these outcomes. Furthermore, placing a euploid embryo increases your chance of success, maximizes your embryo transfers, and hastens your time to a successful pregnancy.

» *Personal Anxiety Regarding Genetic Abnormalities:* Some couples, regardless of age, have significant concerns about genetic disorders or miscarriage and choose IVF with PGT-A to increase their chances of a healthy pregnancy. This is especially true if you have delivered a child with a genetic disease.

- *Excellent Insurance Coverage and Desire for Efficiency:* If you have comprehensive insurance coverage for IVF and wish to expedite the process, IVF is the quickest and most effective route to pregnancy. For some couples, minimizing the time spent trying other less successful methods is a high priority. It's worth noting that many advocate for infertility to be covered by insurance on par with other medical conditions. If you find your coverage lacking, consider voicing your concerns to your human resources department. Regardless of coverage, you can always discuss the option of IVF as a first step with your provider.

In all other scenarios—isolated ovulation disorders, mild male factor infertility, or unexplained infertility—simpler and less expensive treatments first may be a reasonable approach, especially if you lack comprehensive IVF insurance coverage and have a good ovarian reserve (AMH).

Ultimately, the decision of whether to proceed directly to IVF is a personal one that should be made in close consultation with your fertility specialist, taking into account your specific diagnosis, financial considerations, family-building goals, and personal preferences. Don't hesitate to ask questions and advocate for the treatment path that feels right for you.

CHAPTER 11

EMBRACING THE MYSTERIES OF LIFE

Ileft Wake Forest for several reasons, having built their program and served as the IVF director for 16 years. While leaving was tough, I was extremely blessed because my team went with me. We took our program and put it under another healthcare system, and because of my incredible team, were able to start up fairly soon. As I had seen at Vermont University and Wake Forest University, success came quickly. A few years into the new program, I began to hit that season of confidence. I was more efficient and found that patients were very willing to follow my advice. The team was happy and cohesive. Life was good.

Infertility has no boundaries and takes everyone captive. One day I met Marley. She was young, average size, healthy, professional, and seemed to have it all. Yet she suffered from infertility secondary to two factors. First, she didn't ovulate normally. Luckily, ovulation problems are usually easy to fix.

We have excellent fertility drugs that are able to get most of these women pregnant, often with twins and occasionally with triplets. But there was a second factor. Her husband had a meager sperm count. Until the 1990s, these couples often had to turn to donor sperm to achieve a pregnancy. Many adopted because of a hesitation with using sperm from an unknown man.

But in the early 1990s, a physician in Europe discovered how to inject sperm into eggs successfully. A new procedure was born—intracytoplasmic sperm injection (ICSI). And within no time, we began to realize that ICSI brought superb success rates to these couples who in the past had no hope. In other words, with the advent of ICSI, the quality of the sperm became much less important. All of a sudden, all those couples with male problems had another option: IVF with ICSI. New businesses and technologies sprang up to offer the equipment for ICSI. It takes a very sophisticated microscope and needle injection system, but the cost became secondary to the help offered to such a large number of patients. Roughly half of all couples suffer from some type of sperm problem.

When Marley came, the field of ICSI was many years old and very refined. IVF providers soon came to realize that the most important factor, far and away, was the quality of the eggs. All the other problems such as fallopian tube damage, endometriosis, ovulation disorders, and now sperm problems could be overcome with IVF and ICSI.

Another development occurred around 2000 that also revolutionized the field of IVF: blastocyst development. Before the turn of the century, most embryos were transferred back to the uterus three days after fertilization, at the six-to-eight cell stage. The problem is that many day-three embryos are not good quality and either don't implant or lead to miscarriages. Shortly after day three, the embryo changes dramatically. The embryo genome begins to become active, and the cells begin to divide much more rapidly. In just two more days, at day five, it becomes a blastocyst that has more than 100 cells, a cyst cavity, and a group of cells that are programmed by DNA to become the baby, called the inner cell mass. Day-three embryos might look good, but many do not develop into blastocysts, leading to lower success rates with day-three embryo transfers. Blastocysts are much higher quality and implant at a much higher rate. Until the turn of this century, for the first 20 or so years of IVF, no one could successfully grow blastocysts.

The field of IVF has always had an active research component. Thankfully, someone figured out how to successfully grow a blastocyst. Once again, the entire field changed to accommodate this new development. Within no time, the success rate of IVF using a blastocyst transfer was approaching 50% per try. With ICSI and blastocyst development, the majority of women can achieve success as long as there is good egg quality.

In 1978, the year of the first successful IVF birth, there were many factors that made IVF a very complex, surgically based, expensive, and often unsuccessful endeavor. With new techniques such as ICSI and blastocyst development, IVF has become a much simpler office-based, less-costly, and highly successful endeavor. But we must have good eggs because egg quality has become about the only thing that really matters anymore. Good eggs lead to good embryos, which lead to lots of babies.

Back to the story. When Marley and her husband came to see me, I was confident that success was at hand. She was a young woman with good egg quality—it doesn't get any better in the IVF world. And she was also in perfect health, intelligent, and motivated. I felt my confidence peaking. This should be a straightforward case. My team was set in motion to make Marley's dream come true.

Her egg stimulation was a little tricky since she started to hyperstimulate or make too many eggs. That can be dangerous in the field of IVF. But I had cared for many women like her and got her to egg retrieval without too much difficulty. To my delight, I obtained 20 mature eggs from her ovaries. She did well after the retrieval, we obtained a sperm specimen, and our lab director set out to ICSI all the mature eggs. In a typical cycle, 20 mature eggs after ICSI would translate to roughly six or seven day-five embryos, or blastocysts. That many embryos, if frozen in sets of one or two, would give her several separate transfers, each with roughly a 50% chance of success. Giving her the family she so desired seemed easy at this point.

I'll never forget the lab director's words five days after her egg retrieval. "We don't have any blastocysts on Marley." David, my lab director and close friend, was one of the top embryologists in the country. Quiet and confident, he was always one to be trusted. I said "None? Really? How is that even possible? Is there something wrong in the lab?" He replied, "No, all the other patients are doing great and making wonderful blastocysts."

I kept thinking, we know how to do this. We're a very successful program. Zero out of 20 never happens. How do I explain this to Marley? With all our success, even with all my confidence, at that moment I felt like I didn't know anything. Marley trusts us, and I have no answers.

We met Marley and her husband and gave them the unbelievable news. They were confused, and my confidence was waning. I knew we could do better, so we all agreed that something strange must have happened, and the odds were that it would not happen again. So, we embarked on another cycle. She had a great stimulation, and I retrieved 24 mature eggs. The lab director made sure everything in the lab was perfect and the media was just right, and then he focused on her ICSI as intently as he had ever done in the past. And he walked back in my office five days later and once again said we have no blastocysts. How is it possible that 44 eggs from a young woman could lead to no blastocysts? Even with all we know about human fertilization, there was no way to explain this phenomenon.

Marley took the news better this time. Perhaps the first experience had prepared her for this outcome. In fact, she took it like a pro, graciously said her goodbyes, and even thanked us for all the care they had received. They were gone, never realizing how unusual and remarkable their experience truly was.

While we learn confidence through the successful times, we learn humility through the tough times. There's a place for humility, especially in a young doctor's career. With humility comes an understanding that we are not supposed to know everything or be able to fix everyone. With humility, we're more willing to look for answers or seek help from someone else. Confidence is good, but it can lead to risk-taking if we fail to ask for help when needed. While definitely true in medicine, this principle also applies to every aspect of life. We often need help from others.

There comes a time in every young person's career when confidence emerges. Hopefully, it comes at just the right moment, at the intersection of talent and experience. With premature confidence, people can get hurt. With delayed confidence, you can waste a big chunk of your career. As with IVF, timing is everything.

I hope Marley found peace in the midst of her infertility trial. I hope she found contentment and some answers following a very strange occurrence in the world of IVF. And I hope she is now better able to weather seasons of disappointment and transition to a place of contentment. My hope is that her IVF experience, with all its unknowns and strangeness, has prepared her to weather any trial she may face in the future.

She wasn't the only one going through a crisis of confidence. Her cycles taught me some humility and gave me the understanding that there are mysteries in life that we need to embrace. Unanswered questions may be difficult, but they lead you to a humility about life that will serve you well into the future. In short, thanks, Marley.

Dr. Deaton's Prescription: Confidence and humility are companions. Confidence keeps us moving forward, and humility keeps us from running too fast or veering off course. Humility does not mean a lack of confidence or self-respect. A meek and humble person is one with great strength kept in control. It is this strength that spurs hope in us, true hope even in seemingly hopeless situations.

Take a moment to exam yourself. Do you practice humility? And are you keeping hope alive in your life no matter what circumstances you are facing? If someone has helped you practice humility, give them a call and thank them.

How will you follow this prescription?

NAVIGATING DIFFICULT DECISIONS

Donor Eggs, Child-Free Living, and Financial Constraints

Fertility care, particularly IVF, has seen remarkable growth recently due to increased success rates (thanks to advancements such as genetic testing and blastocyst culture) and expanding insurance coverage. It's such a positive trend that many large companies are now including this essential care in their employee benefits. However, let's be honest. These treatments can be expensive, and not all individuals and couples can access them. You might find yourself facing challenging circumstances, and I want to offer some guidance as you navigate these possibilities. How might you approach the following situations if you find yourself in one of these categories?

What if you have good eggs and good sperm, need IVF, but can't afford it? Unfortunately, this is a common and deeply frustrating situation for many. While there are no easy solutions, here are some avenues to consider.

- *Open Communication with Family:* Infertility impacts not just the couple but also their parents and siblings. Sharing your struggles with your family might reveal a willingness to contribute financially to your IVF cycle as it could lead to a cherished grandchild, niece, or nephew. You might be surprised by their support.
- *Explore Refund Programs:* Some fertility programs offer financial packages that provide a significant portion of your money back if treatment is unsuccessful. Carefully review the terms and conditions of these programs as they often require a larger upfront investment. However,

they can offer some financial reassurance, knowing that you will either have a baby (albeit at a higher cost) or recoup a substantial amount of your investment.

• *Strategic Financial Planning:* If your AMH is good and you are younger, time may be on your side. Consider having an open and honest conversation with your partner about your finances and explore ways to gradually save for an IVF attempt. While it's important to continue living your life, perhaps you can identify areas for mindful saving without sacrificing essential needs or occasional joy.

What if you are financially secure and want to do IVF but don't have enough good eggs? This is another common and emotionally challenging scenario. It often brings a profound question to the forefront: How important is it to have a genetic connection with your child? While not inexpensive, it is relatively straightforward to purchase anonymous donor eggs from an established egg bank. These eggs can be fertilized with your partner's sperm, and the resulting embryo can be transferred to your uterus for you to carry. Thankfully, the uterus maintains its ability to support a pregnancy regardless of age. That means you would experience pregnancy, childbirth, and all the joys and responsibilities of parenthood, but your child would not share your genes. How significant is this genetic link for you? Is parenthood fundamentally about genetics? Many would argue it is not.

With a donor egg pregnancy, you will nurture the pregnancy for nine months, your blood will nourish your baby, you will experience the miracle of birth, and you will be the one changing diapers, guiding them through school, and celebrating every milestone. In every meaningful way, you will be their mother. However, you will not be their genetic parent. If the primary desire is to experience motherhood, donor eggs are a viable option. Many couples find peace with this choice as the female partner experiences pregnancy while the male partner provides the sperm, creating a strong bond for both of them with their child. If you are in your 40s or have a very low AMH, discuss donor eggs openly with your provider. It's important to remember that unlike egg quality in women, sperm quality in men typically declines minimally with age.

What if you have great eggs but your partner has no sperm? As discussed earlier, your doctor will likely refer your partner to a Urologist specializing in male infertility. Fortunately, advancements in technology now allow for successful sperm retrieval directly from the testicles, often yielding similar success rates to using ejaculated sperm in IVF. If you have good insurance coverage or are financially secure, you can pursue IVF using testicular sperm. The sperm retrieval procedure, called testicular epididymal sperm extraction (TESE), is often performed in the urologist's office or your fertility specialist's office under local anesthesia with embryologists from the IVF lab present to freeze the retrieved sperm. This testicular sperm can then be thawed and used to fertilize your eggs on the day of retrieval in your fertility specialist's office.

The other option for these couples is to use donor sperm from a reputable sperm bank. In this situation, if the female partner's fertility is otherwise good, simple IUI with donor sperm can lead to high success rates. However, unlike the situation with donor eggs, the female partner provides the egg and carries the child, which can sometimes leave the male partner feeling somewhat disconnected from the pregnancy. It's important to discuss these potential emotional complexities with your doctor, and seeking guidance from a counselor specializing in fertility dilemmas can be very beneficial.

Finally, let's address the important topic of child-free living. We are currently witnessing a significant societal shift with more and more individuals and couples consciously choosing not to have children. This trend, with well over 10% of adults opting for a child-free life, is a significant development. While society will undoubtedly need to adapt to potential shifts in birth rates, this growing acceptance of child-free living is important as it provides future generations with diverse role models and validates a life path that doesn't necessarily include parenthood. While children are often considered a blessing and are the focus of infertility care, there is absolutely nothing wrong with prioritizing career aspirations, friendships, and relationships with nieces and nephews. If you find yourself drawn to the idea of a child-free life, consider speaking with a counselor or seeking advice from others who have made this choice. It's a valid and increasingly common path.

CHAPTER 12

HELP IN A TIME OF GRIEF

After four years of college, four years of medical school, four years of residency, and three more years of infertility training, I felt ready for anything. On one of my early days at Wake Forest in my newly starched white coat, I walked over to the clinic to begin seeing patients—on my own. I was in charge now and didn't have to run my decisions by anyone else. Compared to all my years in training, this day felt like pure freedom—that is, until I pulled the chart out of the slot to go see my very first patient of the day. At that moment, my newfound freedom and confidence took a sudden turn for the worse.

I opened the door while reading the note from Pat, my nurse. The note said, "Patient had her tubes tied and would like another child. About a year ago, her husband came home from work, took their only child out for a treat, and they both died in a terrible car wreck." I was in too far to turn around and walk out, yet I needed to rein in my emotions. Really? I recently finished training. I never had this situation in fellowship, and I have to face this now, unprepared? I wasn't even sure I could make it through the patient evaluation, but I calmed my soul, introduced myself, and began this patient journey as my own man. If only I could hand this off to the "real" doctor as I had done for the past seven years. But there was no one to take the handoff. I was the real doctor.

She was very tall with blonde hair, upper 30s, and had a quiet demeanor about her. Most would say she was grieving and guarded, but I sensed there was more to it. It is sometimes hard to tell the difference between quiet and depressed versus quiet and thoughtful. There seemed to be a depth about her that was hidden by the circumstances of the moment. But I was not her counselor but rather her fertility doctor. I set about doing my job.

We discussed her case and decided to proceed with surgery to reconnect her ligated fallopian tubes. In those days, IVF was not very successful, and she wasn't ready for a child right now. She wanted some more healing. Her psychiatrist believed the surgery and her hope for another child was part of her healing process. I decided to partner with her therapist, and the two of us locked arms to help her. Insurance companies usually deny this type of surgery, so I don't know how she paid for it. While I understand rules are needed to govern insurance coverage, I wish there were easier mechanisms for exceptions to provide the best care for the patient.

I booked the case and moved back from part-time therapist to surgeon. After she was asleep, I made the incision and entered her pelvic cavity. I was distressed to find that one tube was very short. Furthermore, the ovary on the side with the longer, better tube had a large cyst. I paused, realizing that her future mental health might depend on this procedure. Now where was the "real" doctor? Surely someone could come in and do this case for me. Just a short two months ago I would have said to the nurse, "Someone page one of the attending physicians to come and help." But not this time. I was the attending.

I also knew that we don't grow and build character through the easy times, but we grow and develop character through the difficult ones. I took a deep breath, asked for the retractor, started my favorite music (often either Amy Grant or Ella Fitzgerald), and proceeded to remove the cyst and put the ovary back together. I went about reconnecting the good tube on this side. I removed the short tube on the other side with the normal ovary. That left her with no optimal side since the good ovary had no tube, and the surgical ovary had a reconnected tube. I knew this left her with a smaller chance than normal. Two hours later, she was in the recovery room, not realizing that her chance for an ectopic pregnancy was probably around 20% and her chance of a successful birth was about 40%.

The next day, making rounds, I broke the news to her. She took it well, and considering her history of getting bad news, this probably seemed like no big deal to her. I also sensed she was on the road to emotional recovery. She seemed different to me, with a certain quiet confidence rather than a quiet desperation. While they may look similar on the outside, they are polar opposites on the inside. While another baby was an obvious goal, it seemed to me that the courageous act of surgery was a significant part of her healing journey.

During her time in the hospital, I never saw any family members or friends come for a visit. It was no surprise to me; how could she ever open her heart again? She seemed all alone. I would sometimes find her in quiet solitude, lost in her thoughts. Could she get on with her life? Would she always be defined by her incredible loss? I was old enough to know that life can take sudden, unforeseen twists that change someone forever. I had faced my daughter's stillbirth just a few weeks earlier. I knew the devastating feeling of unexpected loss.

But this loss? How can something like this happen? Life is not fair, but having to bury your husband and child at the same time warranted giving up on any fairness in this world. It was easy to understand why some give up on life. Yet even in the midst of such adversity, there are those who are able to rise above it and continue to live, continue to pursue a dream, continue to have more children in spite of insurmountable losses.

On the day of her discharge, I signed the order and went to check her incision and give her discharge instructions. She asked me a question which I will never forget. "Doctor, when I leave the hospital today, is it okay to get on an airplane?" I told her yes and then asked the obvious question: "Where are you going?" At that moment, a man walked into the room to take her away. I introduced myself, and he shook my hand. She said, "I'm moving to Michigan today, and the plane is waiting." I bid her farewell, wishing I could have sent her off with two normal fallopian tubes. But perhaps her new relationship and living a life without children was to be her life's journey. She was strong, and I was confident she would be fine with or without future children. As a fertility physician, I want every woman who wants to get pregnant to get pregnant.

We are designed for interaction. Early in life there is a need for the building of relationships—long conversations into the night, shared interests to discuss, fun activities designed to help us bond with others in important ways. These early friendships give us a foundation for all future relationships. Without this foundation, we can drift into a life of loneliness and despair to a place where there is no margin for adversity. When trials come, as they always do, we need those relationship muscles that allow us to reach out and connect. And if true adversity comes, it may take every ounce of strength to simply ask for help. But help is always around the corner. We just need to ask. She was a living example of these principles.

There are two things she taught me. First, there are times when we face unspeakable grief. The grief process can be quick for some and painstakingly long for others. Grief looks different in every individual. Some cry, some hide, some dive into work, some start a new hobby, and many do all of these. Some never recover from this type of grief, while others refuse to grieve, settling into a life of despair. But this patient was able to come through this grief and embrace a new season of life. She had the courage to start a new relationship, and she dared to trust a young doctor with one of the most important decisions in her life. Her "trust muscles" had been fully developed, probably at a young age.

Second, we need others to help in our time of grief. Much of grief is solitary, but our connections can be the lifeline to provide oxygen when we feel we are under water. We are designed to be in community, not alone. If you're grieving, be open to help that might come onto your path. It may surprise you, but if you have the courage to embrace it, to humble yourself by realizing you can't do it in your own power, you may successfully move into a season of peace and contentment.

Several years went by, and I had not heard from her. I had a full life at work and a full life at home, and over time she slipped from my memory. One day while sitting in my office I opened a card from her with a beautiful picture of twin girls. It remains one of the best cards I have ever received.

Dr. Deaton's Prescription: Grief is a natural and important part of life. But we are not meant to face challenges or grieve alone. We are made to be in relationship. Is there something you are grieving? Have you had the courage to tell someone about it? While grief is important, it is equally important not to get stuck in that grief. At some point, we need to embrace life and move on.

Think of something you have had to grieve. Do you think you are done with the grief process? If not, find someone you trust to confide in. Find someone who can enter into your grief and help you get to the other side.

How will you follow this prescription?

EXPLORING ADOPTION AS ANOTHER OPTION

I recognize that placing this chapter at the end of the book addresses what can be one of the most emotionally challenging crossroads in your infertility journey. Deciding whether to stop pursuing fertility treatments can feel like stepping off a long and demanding emotional roller coaster. If you've been on this path for a significant time without success, you've likely been avoiding this question. But it may be time to gently and honestly consider it.

Let me begin by reiterating a few crucial points.

- *You are in control of your life.* You haven't lost control; you are actively making choices.
- *Infertility is common.* One in seven women under 35 and one in four women between 35 and 40 experience infertility. Many lack insurance coverage or financial means for continued treatment. You are not alone in this experience. Many others, perhaps even those around you, are navigating similar challenges.
- *Your worth is inherent.* Your value as a person is not defined by your ability to conceive and give birth. You are infinitely worthy, regardless of whether you ever deliver a child.
- *Support is available.* Many compassionate individuals can help you navigate this decision, including professionals, trusted friends, family members, and spiritual advisors. While you don't need to share your entire struggle with everyone, confiding in a few trusted individuals can provide invaluable support. Please don't face this difficult time in isolation.

As you contemplate the profound decision of whether to conclude fertility treatments, remember that you will simply be closing one door and opening another to a different and hopefully fulfilling chapter of your life. Grief is a personal process, and everyone navigates it at their own pace. If you have a partner, be mindful that their grieving timeline may differ from yours, which can sometimes create relationship stress. Be patient with each other. When you both feel a sense of peace with your decision, you can confidently step through the next door.

As mentioned earlier, many individuals and couples are now choosing a child-free life. I've witnessed couples make this decision, and after navigating their grief, they often become incredibly loving and involved aunts and uncles. Some couples find deep fulfillment focusing on their careers and their relationship, often achieving greater financial stability and the freedom to pursue other passions. As a fertility specialist, I am not advocating against having children. I simply want to acknowledge the valid and often rewarding aspects of alternative paths.

Regarding having only one child, many couples I work with assume they must provide a sibling for their child, often based on the belief that an only child is somehow disadvantaged. While there are certainly benefits to having siblings, research suggests that an only child is often just as happy and may even achieve greater success in life. In my experience, an only child frequently develops deep and meaningful friendships that can be as enriching as sibling relationships. Please don't feel pressured by the myth that every child must have a sibling.

Having explored the paths of child-free living or having an only child, what if you decide that your journey must involve expanding your family to include more children? If you've exhausted other options discussed in earlier chapters such as donor eggs or donor sperm, adoption may be the next path to consider. There are two main types of adoption I want to discuss: child adoption and embryo adoption.

There are several avenues for individuals and couples to pursue child adoption. One of these may resonate with you, and I hope the following overview helps you begin to explore this new journey.

- *International Adoption:* There are compelling reasons why international adoption might be the right choice for you. It can often be a faster process than domestic adoption due to a larger number of children needing homes. Identifying a reputable agency specializing in international adoptions and focusing on a specific country can also expedite the process. While navigating the unique legal frameworks of different countries can be complex, a dedicated agency will guide you through these intricacies. Moreover, international adoption can broaden your horizons, connecting you with another part of the world and enriching your family in unexpected ways.

- *Private Adoption:* Private adoption presents unique challenges but can offer the opportunity to adopt an American infant, which is often a deeply held desire for couples facing infertility. This type of adoption involves either networking among family, friends, church, and social media to connect with a prospective birth mother or working with an agency specializing in private placements. Finding a birth mother can be challenging, particularly for couples who have kept their infertility struggles private. However, if you are willing to share your story, you might be surprised and deeply moved when a birth mother seeking an adoptive family reaches out and chooses you. It's crucial to be aware that private adoption can also lead to heartbreak if a birth mother changes her mind after delivery, as most states have a grace period allowing her to do so. If you pursue this route, it is essential to hire an experienced adoption attorney who can protect your interests. You can find qualified attorneys through referrals or the American Academy of Adoption Attorneys.

- *Agency Adoption:* While agency adoptions were once the primary route to adoption, they have become less common due to the rise of international and private adoptions. Additionally, many birth mothers today prefer to have more direct involvement in choosing their baby's adoptive parents, leading them away from placing children through agencies. However, if you are open to waiting for a potentially longer period, adopting a healthy infant through an agency can be a safe and relatively less expensive option. It's worth contacting adoption agencies in your area. You might be surprised to learn about children who are currently waiting for families.

- *Special Needs Adoption:* Adopting a child with special needs requires a unique and deeply compassionate heart, but it can also bring immense joy and fulfillment to couples who are eager to share their love with children. Special needs can encompass various situations, including older children (often considered harder to place despite their equal need for loving families), sibling groups (as most people prefer to adopt just one child at a time), and children with disabilities or medical conditions. If you are considering this path, approach it with open eyes, ask thorough questions, and be prepared for a significant commitment that can be profoundly rewarding. Most special needs adoptions are coordinated through local social services departments. Seek their guidance if you feel drawn in this direction as these adoptions often involve unique challenges and require specific support.

Finally, let's discuss embryo adoption. In the United States, most individuals and couples with surplus cryopreserved embryos return to use them for future pregnancies. If they decide not to use their remaining embryos, the majority choose to either donate them to scientific research or discard them. However, a small percentage choose to anonymously donate their embryos to another couple seeking to build a family. Some IVF centers have their own embryo donation programs, while others refer patients to national embryo adoption centers. Many are drawn to embryo adoption as it offers the chance to experience pregnancy and childbirth while also providing an opportunity for unused embryos to develop into life.

While this is a beautiful option, there are a few considerations. First, the number of embryos donated for adoption is relatively small, so finding a good match can take time. Second, assessing the quality of donated embryos can be challenging. However, your fertility provider can offer insights based on the originating IVF center's reputation, the embryos' grading, and any available genetic information. Don't hesitate to inquire about this option at your clinic. Third, embryo adoption can still involve costs, and your financial resources may have been somewhat depleted by your previous fertility treatments. For many couples, embryo adoption offers a final chance at parenthood while also fulfilling a deep desire to give these embryos a chance at life.

CONCLUSION

As you reach the end of this book, it is my sincere hope that you feel a renewed sense of hope and solidarity. The journey through infertility is undeniably arduous, but within the shared experiences and expert guidance offered here lies the powerful reminder that you are not navigating this in isolation. May the stories of resilience ignite your own inner strength, and may the medical insights empower you to make informed decisions with confidence.

Whether your path leads to parenthood or takes a different turn, know that your experience is valid, your feelings are real, and there is profound strength in seeking support and understanding. This book is a testament to the courage and tenacity of the human heart, and it stands as a comforting companion on your unique and deeply personal journey.

www.ingramcontent.com/pod-product-compliance
Lightning Source LLC
Chambersburg PA
CBHW071549200326
41519CB00021BB/6669